'I cann
to read
women

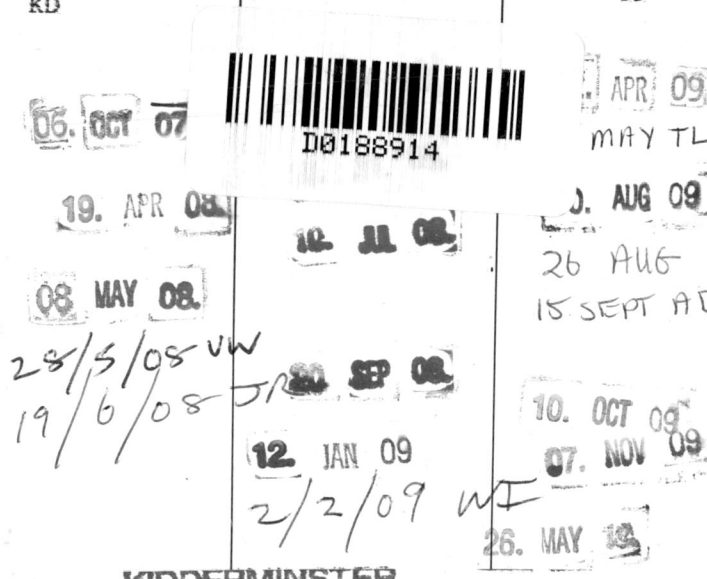

06. OCT 07

19. APR 08

08 MAY 08

28/5/08 VW
19/6/08 JR

APR 09

MAY TL

). AUG 09

26 AUG

15 SEPT AB

12. JAN 09

2/2/09 WT

10. OCT 09

07. NOV 09

26. MAY 19

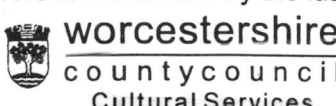

KIDDERMINSTER

11. AUG

FRANCIS-CHEUNG, T.   618.1

The menopause diet: the natural way to
beat your symptoms and lose weight

70003089513   Pbk
Please return/renew this item by the last date shown

worcestershire
countycouncil
Cultural Services

700030895131

The Menopause Diet

The natural way to beat your symptoms
and lose weight

Theresa Cheung with Professor Adam Balen

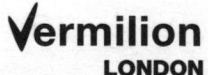

Vermilion
LONDON

1 3 5 7 9 10 8 6 4 2

Published in 2007 by Ebury Publishing

A Random House Group company

Copyright © Theresa Cheung 2007

Theresa Cheung has asserted her right to be identified as the author of this
Work in accordance with the Copyright, Designs and Patents Act 1988

All rights reserved. No part of this publication may be reproduced, stored in
a retrieval system, or transmitted in any form or by any means, electronic,
mechanical, photocopying, recording or otherwise, without the prior
permission of the copyright owner

WORCESTERSHIRE COUNTY COUNCIL	
513	
Bertrams	07.08.07
618.1	£10.99
KD	

The Random House Group Limited Reg. No. 954009

Addresses for companies within the Random House Group can be found at
www.randomhouse.co.uk

A CIP catalogue record for this book is available from the British Library

The Random House Group Limited makes every effort to ensure that the
papers used in our books are made from trees that have been legally sourced
from well-managed and credibly certified forests. Our paper procurement
policy can be found on www.randomhouse.co.uk

Printed in the UK by CPI Mackays, Chatham, ME5 8TD

ISBN 9780091917012

Copies are available at special rates for bulk orders. Contact the sales
development team on 020 7840 8487 or visit www.booksforpromotions.co.uk
for more information.

The advice offered in this book is not intended to be a substitute for the
advice and counsel of your personal physician. Always consult a medical
practitioner before embarking on a diet or a course of exercise. Neither the
author nor the publisher can be held responsible for any loss or claim
arising out of the use, or misuse, of the suggestions made, or the failure to
take medical advice.

Contents

Acknowledgements

I am very grateful to Professor Adam Balen for his commitment to demystifying medical research and for his generous reading of the manuscript, his enthusiastic Foreword and his interest and belief in the book.

A big thank you to Colette Harris for being such an inspiration to work with and to sharing her extensive knowledge of women's health with me.

Special thanks also to my editor Julia Kellaway for her dedication, insight, support, advice, patience and skill.

Finally, special thanks to all the women who spent time talking to me about their concerns about menopause and weight gain – I am truly grateful for the insight they gave me.

Foreword

I cannot recommend this book highly enough. It is easy to read and full of sensible and helpful tips from which all women over the age of 35 will benefit.

It's important to pay attention to lifestyle and diet throughout life but particularly during the menopause. The lowering of circulating oestrogen levels can affect health and wellbeing in a number of ways, as outlined throughout this book. It is, however, an oversimplification to blame declining oestrogen for all these changes. There's certainly evidence that deficiency of other hormones, particularly testosterone, can have a major effect on wellbeing. Using hormone replacement therapy (HRT) to provide the body with sex hormones that are no longer being produced by the ovaries may alleviate some menopausal symptoms, but HRT is also associated with side-effects and potential long-term health risks. Its use has therefore declined significantly in recent years, with more and more women favouring natural alternatives.

The best approach to the menopause is a holistic one. This book presents a highly informed, pragmatic plan with an emphasis on scientifically proven diet and lifestyle therapies. There is helpful advice for all the key areas of concern, from night sweats, irregular periods and insomnia to shifts in weight, mood and libido. The book hits just the right note when considering diet and supplements. This is underpinned by advice on lifestyle and psychological wellbeing. The tips concerning weight gain and how to combat it – an area of particular concern for many women approaching menopause – are sound, sensible and effective.

Punctuated throughout with diet and lifestyle advice to help balance hormones, relieve symptoms and boost quality of life, *The Menopause Diet* is essential reading for all women and their partners and family and should be given a central place in the kitchen and not hidden away on a distant bookshelf.

Adam Balen MD, FRCOG
Professor of Reproductive Medicine and Surgery
Leeds Teaching Hospitals

Introduction

Losing weight is never easy, but once you approach 40 it seems to get harder. The temptation to eat all things sugary is stronger, there's a spare tyre round your belly, and when you try to diet your energy levels drop so much that exercise is definitely off the menu.

It isn't your imagination. Beginning around the age of 35, most women lose about half a pound of muscle and gain one and a half pounds of fat every year; and most of that seems to gather around the waist. This doesn't sound like too much but after five years and seven pounds, then perhaps 10 years and 15 pounds, it can really start to add up.

Don't blame yourself – blame biology, blame the pace of modern life. A number of pesky factors – such as a slowing metabolism, the constant daily menace of stress and decreasing oestrogen levels associated with menopause – all seem to be stacking the odds against you. Although it is harder to lose weight, don't worry – it's *not* impossible. What you need is an easy-to-follow plan that doesn't leave you hungry or with a sluggish metabolism, and that doesn't age you by starving your body of nutrients that can keep your skin smooth and your belly firm. That's where this book comes in. Just when you thought you'd never get the same weight-loss results, it offers the very latest research into the causes of midlife weight gain and new and effective solutions.

So, if you're over 35 and concerned about your weight and/or your willpower, *The Menopause Diet* has been written for you. You'll discover that by making simple changes to your diet and the way you eat it's possible to maintain or lose weight and feel good about yourself. And while you're dropping a dress size or two you'll also be boosting your energy and libido, reducing your risk of osteoporosis, heart disease, diabetes and cancer, and increasing your chances of living longer. Not bad side-effects of whittling down your waist!

A Healthier, Slimmer, Happier You

Studies on diets eaten by the world's healthiest women – the Japanese – show that menopausal symptoms and the possibility of weight gain can be largely eliminated through simple diet and lifestyle choices. *The Menopause Diet* is based on this research. It covers the foods you need to eat before, during and after menopause to ease your symptoms and lose weight. The foods are really easy to incorporate into your daily meals, and the whole family can eat them.

It often helps to know that you aren't alone. In this book you'll learn about the latest research into the bodily changes all women face and why we're more likely to gain weight in the run-up to the menopause, especially around the middle. If you feel ready to dive right in, you can head straight to Chapter 3, 'The Menopause Diet' and Chapter 4, 'The Menopause Diet Detox Boost'. The advice given in these chapters is based on cutting-edge research into the causes of menopause weight gain and offers effective solutions. It will give you the foundation you need to work through the rest of the book and create a weight-loss plan that works for you and your specific symptoms. If you're worried you won't be able to stay the course, there's also plenty of advice about how you can stay motivated when the going gets tough, and how there's so much to look forward to, whatever your age or stage in life.

Although your mother or grandmother may have used the term 'the change' to refer to the menopause, it isn't a single event. Instead, it's a transition that can start in your 30s or 40s and last into your 50s or even 60s, and you may begin to experience signs and symptoms of menopause well before your periods stop permanently.

Whether you are in your 30s or your 60s, *The Menopause Diet* will be your guide to navigating the hormonal changes and metabolism shifts that can trigger symptoms such as weight gain, night sweats, loss of libido, insomnia and mood swings. With this plan, nothing can stop you losing weight and feeling healthier, happier and sexier than ever.

The HRT Dilemma

Should you take hormone replacement therapy (HRT)? That's a question every woman has to face sooner or later. The information below should help you make up your mind.

What is HRT?

Millions of women throughout the world take hormone replacement therapy to ease the symptoms of menopause and to protect against menopause-related health risks such as osteoporosis.

HRT does what its name suggests: it replaces the ovarian hormones, oestrogen and progesterone, that are no longer produced when the ovaries cease to function at menopause. It can be started at any age but is most often prescribed at menopause and taken for around five years to control symptoms such as hot flushes and night sweats. HRT can be taken by pill, cream or patch, and the hormone dosage can be raised or lowered according to your personal circumstances and the severity of your symptoms.

HRT: the pros

- HRT is an effective treatment for the symptoms of oestrogen deficiency, including hot flushes, night sweats, vaginal dryness and urinary incontinence. (Hot flushes and night sweats tend to improve after a few weeks of treatment. Vaginal dryness takes a little longer to respond but eventually often does.)
- HRT also reduces the risk of osteoporosis and heart disease associated with oestrogen deficiency.
- HRT is thought to be particularly helpful and safe for women who experience menopause before the age of 40 to reduce their increased risk of osteoporosis and heart disease.
- Increasing evidence also indicates that HRT can reduce the symptoms of arthritis and the risk of colorectal cancer.

HRT: the cons

- Recent studies have shown an increasing risk of breast cancer associated with the use of HRT.
- There may also be an increased risk of stroke and thrombosis (blood clots in the veins).
- Some studies suggest a link between HRT and ovarian and endometrial cancer.
- Another finding has questioned the benefit of HRT for the prevention of heart disease and strokes.

It's important, though, to put the health risks of HRT in perspective as most women on HRT do not experience these problems, and other risk factors such as being overweight and smoking are also to blame.

Side-effects of HRT

Around 35 per cent of women stop taking HRT because of unwanted side-effects. These can often be resolved by a change in the dose or type of HRT so it's important to discuss any problems with your doctor before deciding to stop.

The most commonly reported side-effects of oestrogen include fluid retention, bloating, breast tenderness and cramps, nausea and stomach upsets. The side-effects of progesterone include fluid retention, breast tenderness, depression, nausea, irritability, mood swings, abdominal pain, backache and acne. Most side-effects disappear within the first two to three months of taking HRT.

Many women are concerned that HRT will make them put on weight, but various studies prove that weight gain is not linked to hormone therapy. If a woman is prone to weight gain during her middle years, this will happen regardless of her HRT use. A few women may be sensitive to oral oestrogen, particularly if the dose is too high, causing them to retain fluid and gain weight. Simply reducing the dose or changing to a non oral form can resolve this.

So where does all this leave women considering or taking HRT? Barely a month goes by without HRT and its possible risks hitting the headlines, but as things stand researchers believe there are very few risks associated with short-term use for women starting to take it around the age of 50. However, we still don't know the risks and benefits if the same women decide to take it for more than five years. Nor do we really know the best type or dose of HRT to take.

Making your mind up

Using HRT is neither right nor wrong. You must, in consultation with your doctor, weigh up the pros and cons and decide what works best for you. Never forget that you do have options. If you're finding it difficult to tolerate the side-effects of HRT, or if it isn't helping your symptoms, ask your doctor about your options. If you don't need or want to take HRT or non-HRT drugs of any kind, you may want to discuss the natural approach with your doctor.

If you decide against HRT, follow the Menopause Diet guidelines and take the recommended supplements. If you're experiencing menopausal symptoms, take the herbs and supplements recommended in Chapter 7 and add in other supplements that might be useful to you.

Natural HRT

If diet and lifestyle changes don't ease your symptoms, another option to consider is natural HRT. Sometimes known as bio identical HRT, natural HRT is made from natural plant sources such as soya, and chemically processed into an oestrogen that's identical to the sort your body makes. Studies show this mixture can be safer and more protective of breast tissue than conventional HRT but it can still have side-effects such as bloating and headaches.

Very few doctors offer natural HRT. Many, however, are starting to take an interest in complementary medicines and doing extra training so you never know – yours might be a qualified herbalist. If not, seek advice from a professional herbalist who will be able to prescribe the right remedy and dosage for you.

Stopping HRT

If you are taking HRT and want to stop you need to speak to your doctor. They may give you a lower dosage of the same drug or change your drug to reduce any side effects you may be suffering from. If you are determined to stop, do so gradually over a period of three months, taking a lower and lower dose if possible. During this three-month period, really work on the Menopause Diet guidelines, start taking supplements and begin a good exercise programme. At the end of the three months you can use herbs if you are getting hot flushes and other symptoms.

If you are taking HRT and it's working properly you shouldn't need any supplementary herbs. Although you can skip the section on herbs, you are strongly advised to follow the Menopause Diet and lifestyle guidelines. They will do you and your waistline nothing but good and protect you naturally against other conditions like heart disease, osteoporosis and cancer. If you still want to take herbs talk to your doctor as certain herbs may interact with HRT.

Time for a Change

Whether or not you decide to opt for HRT, research has shown that you can literally eat your way through the menopause to a healthier, slimmer and happier life. So if you are ready to defy time, hormones and gravity, the Menopause Diet really is the only diet plan you'll ever need. In just a few weeks you'll be on your way to shedding symptoms, pounds, years and worries.

It's time for a change. Leave the fad diet frustrations and stress to others. This highly enjoyable and satisfying diet and lifestyle plan is made for you.

What is the Menopause?

If you're worried about what's going to happen to your body as you round the corner of 40 years it can help to know that you're not alone. *All* women face the same biological changes, so before looking more closely at ways to tackle stubborn midlife weight gain, let's give you the lowdown on what your body is going through.

One Day in Your Life

First of all, the term menopause actually refers to only one day in your life: the 365th day from the date of your last period. Many women have plenty of false starts and may go for months without a period before getting one.

The 365th day is important because it means your body is no longer producing enough of the hormone oestrogen that regulates your menstrual cycle. Oestrogen deficiency is a gradual process that takes place several years before the menopause. The average age of menopause for women in the West is 51 but the normal range is between 46 and 54. Some women reach the menopause in their 30s and a few in their 60s. About half of all women stop menstruating before 51 and about half afterwards. Don't panic if your periods stop before you hit 45 as this happens to about a third of all women, and if you're still menstruating in your

50s this is normal too. (*See also, 'Can I Predict My Last Period?', page 14.*)

What Causes the Menopause?

Your ovaries trigger menopause because their life span is 40 or so years shorter than yours. You depend on your ovaries to produce most of the oestrogen in your body, as well as the other two important sex hormones: progesterone and androgen. Oestrogen and progesterone regulate your periods and androgen fuels your sex drive.

The production of oestrogen and progesterone in your ovaries depends on a complex interaction with other hormones, in particular follicle stimulating hormone (FSH) and luteinizing hormone (LH) secreted by your pituitary gland. Hormone production also depends on the ability of your ovaries to mature and release an egg, because while an egg is maturing it produces oestrogen, and when it is released after ovulation the empty egg sac, called the corpus luteum, produces progesterone.

Menopause occurs when your ovaries run out of functioning eggs. At the time of birth, you had about one to three million eggs, which are gradually lost as you get older. By the time of your first menstrual period, you had an average of 400,000 eggs. By the time of menopause, you may have fewer than 10,000 eggs. A small percentage of these eggs is lost through normal ovulation (the monthly cycle) but most eggs die off through a process called atresia. As you head towards your 40s your ovaries don't respond so well to FSH and LH, and levels of these hormones rise. You'll have fewer cycles in which you ovulate, and because progesterone is produced after ovulation there is typically a drop-off in progesterone first. Finally, when there are no more eggs left, your ovaries make smaller and smaller amounts of oestrogen and then stop working altogether.

The gradual loss of oestrogen during menopause is believed to be the cause of many of the associated symptoms, such as irregular periods, hot flushes, disrupted sleep, night sweats, headaches, vaginal dryness, dry skin and mood swings. This is because oestrogen doesn't just regulate your periods; it also affects many parts of your body, including the blood vessels, heart, bones, breasts, uterus, urinary system, skin and brain. After menopause, your ovaries also decrease their production of testosterone, a hormone involved in libido or sexual drive, and this can cause a dip in your sex drive.

Peri What?

The term perimenopause is a recent one. It simply means around or near the menopause, say around eight years or so before menopause and about a year after. So for most of us perimenopause begins in the early 40s but it can start as early as 35.

Perimenopause is a time of fairly subtle hormonal changes that start to become more obvious as you approach menopause. If you have any health conditions such as premenstrual syndrome (PMS), irregular periods or migraines, you may find these are aggravated by your unstable hormones. You may have your first hot flush or night sweat during this time and find yourself saying, 'Is it hot in here or is it just me?' You may also feel tired and find it hard to concentrate or feel irritable or anxious for no reason. In short, you may just not feel right. It's important to give yourself a break if you do feel wobbly now and again. Oestrogen, remember, affects all parts of your body, and even your brain feels deprived if it doesn't get the fix it's expecting.

Are You in Perimenopause?

If you tick five or more of the following symptoms, the chances are you are in perimenopause.

- Have your periods changed? Have they become irregular or has your cycle got shorter?
- Just before your period, are you irritable and bloated and do you crave sweet foods?
- Are you getting more headaches?
- Are you finding it hard to sleep?
- Have you had any hot flushes or night sweats?
- Are you having mood swings?
- Do you have frequent memory lapses?
- Have you noticed a reduction in vaginal secretions?
- Have you noticed that your hair is less thick?
- Is your skin drier, more sensitive or spot prone?

During perimenopause and approaching menopause, periods may occur more often, the flow may be lighter or heavier, or you may begin to skip periods. It's important to bear in mind that irregular periods might be symptoms of other conditions such as thyroid problems, fibroids, severe PMS or polycystic ovary syndrome (PCOS), so it's always worth visiting your doctor to rule out serious health problems.

For most of us, perimenopause is a tougher ride than menopause and life beyond. Fortunately, the diet and lifestyle changes recommended in this book will help you and your body adjust to lower levels of oestrogen so that your symptoms subside. In the meantime, if you are having a rough time with a certain symptom or symptoms, have a look at Chapter 8: Menopause SOS.

Are There Tests for Menopause?

A visit to your doctor may help determine if you are in perimenopause. He or she will rule out pregnancy and take a blood test to check your oestrogen levels. The most reliable test is to measure your FSH (follicle stimulating hormone), a hormone produced by the pituitary gland to stimulate oestrogen production. As the ovaries' production of oestrogen decreases, levels of FSH increase. Levels of 30 to 40miU/ml (milli international units per millilitre) or above could mean you are in perimenopause. Levels from 10 to 30 mean there is still partial ovarian function. Bear in mind, however, that the test isn't completely foolproof because FSH levels tend to fluctuate a lot during perimenopause and can be misleading. If you prefer not to visit your doctor, home-testing menopause kits are now available at your chemist or over the internet, although they are not as reliable as a visit to your doctor.

What if I'm on the Pill?

Taking the combined contraceptive pill may mask the perimenopause by controlling symptoms such as irregular periods, hot flushes and night sweats. Therefore, it may be difficult to assess when you are no longer fertile. Your doctor can carry out the blood test described above to measure levels of oestrogen and FSH, but this should be planned for the last day of the pill-free interval. Taking the combined contraceptive pill doesn't change the time of your menopause, but withdrawal bleeds will continue for however long you take the pill.

The combined pill can be taken until the menopause if you are healthy and a non-smoker. However, it shouldn't be taken if you are a smoker aged over 35. The progestogen-only pills (POPs) can be taken until the menopause if you are a smoker. However, as they do not contain oestrogen, they will not control or mask any perimenopausal symptoms.

Too Young for All This?

Menopause before the age of 40 is called premature ovarian failure. About 1 per cent of women go through menopause early and it tends to run in families. Tests show that the cause may be an immune response to the body's own ovarian tissue. There may also be an association between premature ovarian failure and other autoimmune disorders, such as type one diabetes and thyroiditis (inflamed thyroid gland). Smoking also increases the risk of an early menopause. If you are in your 30s and experiencing symptoms of menopause you should visit your doctor to get your oestrogen and FSH levels measured and other serious medical conditions ruled out.

Can I Predict My Last Period?

You can't tell when you'll have your last period but there are some factors that will influence its timing. The age you started menstruating may affect the age you experience menopause, although no studies have yet proved this. It's possible, too, that the age your mother experienced menopause will be relevant, although again there's no scientific proof. Women with autumn birthdays may have a later menopause than those born in springtime. Preliminary research has shown that women born in March reached an average menopause age of 48 while those born in October reached it aged 50. Something else to blame your mother for!

Overweight women tend to have a later menopause because body fat can convert some hormone precursors into oestrogen, although the higher oestrogen level puts them at increased risk of breast cancer. Thinner women tend to have a rougher ride with their symptoms during menopause and are at higher risk of osteoporosis than women with some extra body fat. Poor diet, lack of exercise and smoking can also increase the likelihood of an early menopause.

Finally, two factors that *don't* influence menopause are whether you are taking the contraceptive pill or the age at which you had your first or last child.

How Long Will I Stay Fertile?

Between peak childbearing years and menopause, a woman's fertility gradually declines, reducing her risk of an unplanned pregnancy. Yet, a risk still exists. If you don't want to get pregnant, you therefore need to use contraception during perimenopause, and you should continue to use it until you haven't had a period or any bleeding for two years if aged under 50, and for one year if over 50.

Major Health Risks Associated with Menopause

Breast cancer

Roughly one in every 50 women over the age of 50 is affected by breast cancer. While the risk rises steadily throughout a woman's reproductive years, it increases even more following menopause when levels of oestrogen without progesterone to balance them may cause cells in the breast to become cancerous (*see 'What Causes the Menopause?', page 10*). Other risk factors include:

- family history
- excess weight
- poor diet
- early menstruation (before age 12)
- late menopause (after age 55)
- having a first child after the age of 30
- never having children

Hormone replacement therapy (HRT) may increase this risk. Your best protection is to eat healthily, exercise regularly, watch your weight and catch any warning signs early by faithfully performing monthly breast self-examinations and having regular mammograms. A mammogram can spot cancer up to two years before you or your doctor would be able to feel a lump. Talk to your doctor about when you should begin having mammograms, and how often to have them. (*See also the tips on how to examine your breasts on page 161.*)

Heart disease

Many women are surprised to learn that heart disease is the leading cause of death among post-menopausal women. In fact, women are 12 times more likely to die from heart disease than breast cancer. Recent studies show that hormone replacement therapy (HRT) doesn't protect against heart disease and may, in fact, slightly increase the risk of heart attacks, strokes and blood clots. If you are considering HRT, be sure to discuss this risk with your doctor.

Other factors that can increase your likelihood of developing heart disease include:

- ageing
- being menopausal/post-menopausal
- family history
- smoking
- lack of exercise and/or being overweight
- diabetes
- high cholesterol
- high blood pressure
- heavy alcohol consumption

There are many things you can do to prevent and/or lower your risk of heart disease. Discuss these suggestions with your doctor who can set you on the path to good heart health for years to come by recommending some or all of the following:

- stop smoking
- treat high blood pressure
- reduce your cholesterol
- control your weight
- exercise
- enjoy a high-fibre diet
- include more soya in your diet
- enjoy alcohol in moderation
- keep stress under control
- utilise aspirin therapy (*see also Chapter 8, page 213*)

As mentioned earlier, HRT can increase the risk of heart disease and breast cancer, so please discuss this with your doctor.

Osteoporosis
This common health risk is directly linked to the post-menopausal years when lack of oestrogen causes the cells that build new bone to be less active than cells that remove old bone. In other words, your bones are being torn down faster than they are being built up. The excessive loss of bone mass causes osteoporosis, a thinning and weakening of the bones. Osteoporosis increases your risk of a fracture and can lead to a loss of height and/or a humped back.

This disease comes on silently; there are no warning signs and it isn't usually detected until a fracture is suffered. It moves quickly with up to 20 per cent of expected lifetime bone loss occurring within the first five to seven years after the menopause. The good news is that osteoporosis is highly preventable and treatable. There are steps you can take to look after your bones, such as regular exercise and including calcium-rich foods in your diet. (*For more advice and tips on prevention, see Chapter 8, page 206.*)

Life after Menopause

When you've had 365 days without a period you're considered to be in the post-menopausal phase of your life. Your ovaries are no longer producing enough oestrogen and progesterone to support ovulation and menstruation.

Far from seeing life after menopause as the beginning of the end, many women today see it as a new beginning. Study after study has shown that many of us feel the post-menopausal years to be the best time of our lives – a turning point even – when we have more time and energy to focus on career, relationships, sex, interests, hobbies and ourselves.

As far as your symptoms are concerned, after menopause you'll find that they gradually fade away but there will be physical changes to contend with as a result of hormonal change and ageing. The mucous membranes of the vagina become thinner and drier which can make sex and urination painful. You may experience thinning of the skin as well as raised cholesterol levels. Your bone mass and muscle tone may also shrink, especially if you don't exercise. If this sounds really shocking, bear in mind that these changes can take years, even decades, to appear. They are also easy to treat, even prevent, with diet and lifestyle change and, if absolutely necessary, drugs.

The aim of this book isn't just to help you manage your weight; it's also to give you the tools you need to sail through every stage of your menopause – before, during and after – feeling fitter, healthier, slimmer and sexier than ever.

Midlife Expansion

Noticing a few extra pounds around your waist lately? Welcome to midlife expansion, the body change that plagues women between the ages of 35 and 55.

You might find that your weight increases and you have difficulty keeping the extra pounds off. Don't worry – you're not alone. Most women gain around 10 to 15 pounds during their perimenopausal years, and the weight gain is sneaky and gradual – about a pound a year. (Women who have experienced early menopause or surgical menopause may experience more rapid and extreme weight gain.) You may also discover that your body shape is different and your weight isn't distributing itself as it used to.

Your Changing Shape

Many women complain about a softening around the waist as menopause approaches. Despite their best efforts at weight control, the pounds start to creep on around the abdomen, instead of around the hips, thighs and bottom. Women become 'apple shaped' as the stomach becomes rounder. Suddenly, skirts or trousers with elastic waistbands seem a great idea!

Not only does a thickening waist look and feel uncomfortable, it's also bad news for your health, according to a 25-year study at Gothenburg University in Sweden. No one is really sure why being an apple carries more health risks than a pear but it may be due to the way the body processes fat stored in different areas. Fat around the tummy is constantly being broken down and circulated around the body, while fat around the bottom is not. Higher levels of circulating fat increase the risk of heart disease and narrowing of the arteries. Abdominal fat can also put pressure on internal organs, especially the heart.

The spare tyre problem, and the health risks it brings, is a great incentive for keeping to a healthy weight during menopause. However, even if you are careful about what you eat, losing weight has never seemed more difficult. For the first time in your life it may be hard for you to shed a few unwanted pounds. You may be eating and exercising in exactly the same way as you always have, but the weight just refuses to budge. Research now shows that weight gain during menopause is influenced by shifting hormones and a number of other factors, not just lack of willpower.

Hormones and Weight Maintenance

Your body's hormones have a direct impact on your appetite, metabolism and fat storage. This is why it's so difficult to control your weight during menopause: no matter what you do, fluctuating oestrogen, testosterone and androgen levels will fight you all the way.

Oestrogen

No concrete evidence exists that a deficiency of oestrogen causes body fat to accumulate but it does seem that oestrogen may affect the activity of your fat cells and influence body fat distribution around your stomach. One theory is that as your ovaries produce less oestrogen, your body looks for other places to get needed oestrogen from. Fat cells in your body can produce oestrogen, so your body works harder to convert calories into fat to increase oestrogen levels. Unfortunately for you, fat cells don't burn calories the way muscle cells do, which causes you to pack on the unwanted pounds.

Declining levels of oestrogen may also have an impact on your appetite. More studies are needed but it appears that as oestrogen production decreases, your appetite increases because oestrogen suppresses appetite. Now that's something to chew over.

Progesterone

During menopause, progesterone levels will also decrease. Like oestrogen, lower levels of this hormone can be responsible for many of the symptoms of menopause including weight gain, or at least the appearance of it. Water retention, bloating and menopause often go hand in hand due to decreased progesterone levels. Although this doesn't actually result in weight gain, your clothes will probably feel a lot tighter.

Androgen

This hormone is responsible for sending weight gain directly to your middle section. During the menopausal years, weight gain is often known as middle-age spread because of the rapid growth of the midriff. Androgen hormone (like testosterone, which is an androgen hormone) helps your body to create lean muscle mass out of the calories you take in. Muscle cells burn more calories than fat cells do, increasing your metabolism. In menopause, levels of androgen drop gradually, resulting in the loss of this muscle mass. Unfortunately, this lowers your metabolism, which means your body burns calories more slowly and you pile on the pounds.

Other Factors in Midlife Weight Gain

Hormonal changes associated with menopause aren't necessarily the only cause or trigger of weight gain. Ageing and lifestyle factors also play a big role, as detailed below.

Insulin resistance

Problems with blood sugar are a frequent cause of weight gain after the age of 40. Insulin is the hormone that stabilises blood sugar levels, metabolism and your weight. Most women with an eye on their figure follow a low-fat, high-carbohydrate diet, but after a while the wrong kinds of carbohydrates – particularly processed and refined ones loaded with sugar – may make the body resistant to insulin produced in the bloodstream. When this happens the calories you take in quickly turn to fat.

Exercising less

There is a tendency in some women over the age of 35 to exercise less than other women, and this can lead to weight gain. In fact, the most common cause of weight gain at any age is inactivity.

Poor eating habits

Eating foods low in nutrients means you'll take in empty calories. These are converted to fat if you don't burn them for energy.

Burning fewer calories

The number of calories you need decreases slightly as you age because ageing promotes the replacement of muscle with fat. Muscle burns more calories than fat does. When your body composition shifts to more fat and less muscle, your metabolism slows down.

In the family

Genetic factors may play a role in weight gain as well. If your parents and other close relatives carry extra weight around the abdomen, you may be predisposed to do so too. Don't use this as an excuse though! Whether or not your relatives are overweight, weight gain is certainly not inevitable and there is plenty you can do to fight the flab and this book shows you how.

Stress

Poor sleeping habits and stress can also contribute to a thickening waistline. (*For more information on the damaging effects of stress, see Chapter 4.*)

Protecting Your Future Health

If you're approaching menopause, excess weight doesn't just make it hard for you to put on your jeans; it also carries with it serious health risks. The key hormone involved is oestrogen.

Oestrogen is produced by your ovaries, the adrenal glands (that sit on top of the kidneys) and your body fat. Fat produces oestrogen all your life, and this is one of the reasons why a very low-fat diet is such bad news for women. In the right amounts, oestrogen protects your bones and your heart, but problems occur if levels rise too high or fall too low. If you don't have enough oestrogen your bones and heart are at risk, but if you have too much you risk cancer and diabetes.

Because body fat manufactures oestrogen, the more overweight you are the more oestrogen you're likely to have. That's why it's fine to carry a few extra pounds at menopause since this extra oestrogen will balance out the oestrogen decline from the ovaries. If you are very overweight, however, the excess oestrogen can increase your risk of breast and womb cancer because cancer cells in these areas are stimulated by oestrogen. Other conditions influenced by high oestrogen levels include endometriosis (when the lining of the womb grows outside the womb), fibroids (benign tumours in the womb), heavy periods and tender, sore breasts.

One of the simplest and most effective ways to balance your oestrogen levels is to eat healthily. Eating right can not only help you balance your hormones, manage your weight and deal with the day-to-day reality of your symptoms, it can also protect your future health and prolong your life.

Why Diets Don't Work

With excess weight, particularly around the waist, putting a strain on your jeans, your heart and your health, the answer is simple: keep to a healthy weight. So is dieting the answer? Absolutely not!

Dieting to lose weight during perimenopause is perhaps the worst thing you can do. You may see a quick weight loss in the first few weeks but this is actually calorie-burning muscle and water. In the long run you just gain all the weight back with nothing to show for it but saggy skin.

The first reason diets don't work is that restricting your food intake or calorie counting sends a message to your body to go into storage mode. This is referred to as the 'famine effect': your body, thinking it won't get food again for a long time, slows your metabolism and stores every calorie it takes in, causing weight gain. Diets don't work at the best of times, and they're spectacularly unsuccessful during the menopausal transition when you need to be speeding up your metabolism, not slowing it down.

The second reason diets fail is that many fad diets restrict your intake of nutrients, and when you're trying to lose weight you need all the nutrients you can get. For example, if you're eating a high-protein diet you won't be getting the nutrients you need from complex carbohydrates, such as brown rice, which can give you energy, lift your mood, burn calories and boost your sex drive.

An adequate intake of nutrients from all food groups is essential to your health and wellbeing. This is because food is fuel. It helps your body function at optimum levels. Scrimp on the quality and quantity and you pay the price. If you aren't eating well this can unsettle your hormones, compromise your immune system and make you more susceptible to weight gain, colds and infections. You may also be at greater risk of developing health conditions such as heart disease, cancer, diabetes, irregular periods, hypertension, depression, stress, insomnia, arthritis and osteoporosis.

The Menopause Diet isn't about restricting your food choices or starving yourself of nutrients. Rather, it's about eating lots of healthy foods to ease your symptoms and boost your metabolism so the extra weight melts away. In short, it's about eating more, not less. It's a diet of plenty.

Get the Balance Right

Before you plunge in with the Menopause Diet, it's important to keep in mind that a little weight gain as you age is normal and to be expected. There are three times in a woman's life when weight gain is normal and healthy: puberty, pregnancy and menopause. About 90 per cent of menopausal women will gain a little weight between the ages of 35 and 55.

It may be difficult, especially if you've kept a close eye on your weight all your life, but it's important to learn to accept menopause and perhaps the few extra pounds it brings as something natural and even beneficial. Slim is good but too thin at menopause isn't. As we have seen, your body needs some fat to manufacture oestrogen, and if your oestrogen drops too low you are more likely to suffer menopausal symptoms, such as hot flushes and mood swings. Not only can a little extra weight ease symptoms associated with menopause, it also protects you against lady-killers like osteoporosis.

Instead of hating your body, try to be more accepting of yourself. This doesn't mean you should pile on the pounds and forget about ever wearing tight jeans again; it just means you should get a sense of balance and perspective. Gaining too much weight certainly isn't healthy and can be extremely damaging to your health; but on the other hand it isn't the end of the world if you go up one dress size or are a few pounds curvier than you were when you were 20. The important thing is to feel fit and healthy.

Having said all that, if you feel uncomfortable about the prospect of menopause weight gain there are steps you can take to prevent it before it starts. And if you've already begun adding a little too much to your waistline or have gone up a few too many dress sizes, it's never too late to change course with the Menopause Diet.

The Menopause Diet

You may find that a change in diet is all you need to manage your weight, ease your symptoms and reduce the long-term health risks of menopause; or you may decide to talk to your doctor about hormone replacement therapy. Whatever you decide to do, a good diet and nutritional programme is the essential foundation – in partnership with exercise – for the management of menopause, regardless of any additional medicines, herbs or treatments you may use.

Your Daily Dose of Self-help on a Plate

The symptoms of menopause can often batter your self-esteem and make you feel low and depressed. Taking charge of your diet can transform your feelings of helplessness into a more positive attitude because it's something *you* can take control of every day. The lift you get from doing something to ease your symptoms and boost your energy can be really motivating.

Changing your eating habits may seem like a daunting challenge right now but the Menopause Diet isn't complicated, time-consuming or unsatisfying. All you need to do to ease your symptoms and kick-start permanent weight loss is to follow the easy guidelines that follow and start making healthy food choices today. Nothing could be simpler.

The following 10 steps focus on one aspect of the Meno-pause Diet at a time. For each step an explanation is given as to why the recommended dietary change is so beneficial if you're approaching or experiencing menopause, and how it will affect your body and your health.

The steps are arranged in an order that makes for the easiest way to start introducing changes to your life. Try each change and stick with it for a couple of days or however long you need to feel comfortable before moving on to the next step. Be sure to give yourself time to adjust to the diet. If you're used to eating a certain way, it will take time to re-educate your taste buds. It typically takes most people a month or two to adjust to a new eating plan.

Step One: Forget about Dieting

Although this is the Menopause Diet, it isn't really a diet. It's a healthy-eating plan that will encourage you to eat fresh, healthy and delicious foods to help you lose weight and feel great.

The word 'diet' suggests something that has a beginning and an end; a quick fix, not a way of life. It also implies that the weight will pile back on as soon as you stop the diet. You may have been following one diet or another for much of your life, or spent years worrying about how to lose weight. But if your goal is health and happiness rather than weight loss, your whole relationship with food will change. The diet mentality is a hard one to break, especially if the pounds have been piling on, but when you start thinking about food as a way to protect your health and boost your energy something amazing starts to happen. You lose weight without even trying!

Take action

* **Enjoy your food.** You really are what you eat. What you

put into your mouth will affect how you look, think and feel – but don't let this intimidate you. Healthy eating should never take the enjoyment out of eating and deprive you of all the tastes and foods you love. Eat a wide variety of foods and don't cut any food groups out. Have fun filling your plate with colour and experimenting with all the fresh, healthy, delicious and satisfying tastes and food choices out there.

- **Follow the 80/20 rule:** stick to the Menopause Diet guidelines 80 per cent of the time and treat yourself for the other 20 per cent. You can't eat healthily all the time, and the occasional indulgence isn't going to hurt you and doesn't mean you've failed; it's the excesses that count. That way you really can have your cake and eat it.

- **If you have a difficult relationship with food** or are prone to comfort eating, refer to the advice in Chapter 6 before beginning the Menopause Diet.

- **Ditch the diet foods.** Diet foods might be low in fat but they're often lacking in nutrition and packed with sugar. Excess sugar means you get blood sugar swings that spark food cravings; it gives you wrinkles (sugar disrupts our skin's collagen production) and increases your risk of health problems like insulin resistance and diabetes. On top of all that, diet foods with additives and sweeteners may even make you overeat. This is because giving your body something that tastes like it has a lot of calories but doesn't makes you more likely to crave high-calorie foods. So don't load your basket with fat-free foods – you're better off enjoying one full-fat biscuit than stuffing down five diet ones for the same number of calories.

- **Think of the Menopause Diet as a guide to a lifetime of healthy eating.** You can use it to ensure your body gets all the nutrients it needs to ease your symptoms and give you radiant skin, strong bones and boundless energy. Your weight loss will be a by-product of the healthier and happier you.

Step Two: Eat More Often

Ignore your mum's advice not to eat between meals. The Menopause Diet is about eating more, not less, as long as those foods are healthy and nutritious. It's also about eating more often. Try not to go more than three or four hours without eating. Many of us find ourselves skipping breakfast or grabbing a coffee, followed by a light lunch and then an evening meal that can be as late as 9 or 10pm. Starving and stacking your calories like this just isn't a good idea.

Going for long periods without food can encourage weight gain (see 'Why Diets Don't Work', page 24). Skipping meals may slow your metabolism (fat burning) by as much as 5 per cent but eating regular meals and snacks every few hours keeps your metabolism purring along because your stomach is never empty. Long gaps between meals also create low blood sugar levels that make you crave high-calorie foods and snacks – the very foods that contribute to weight gain. A healthy snack between meals, on the other hand, reminds your body that you have a regular supply of food so it won't go into starvation mode and slow your metabolism. It also helps you lose weight by keeping your blood sugar levels steady, which in turns helps to keep your moods and your hormone levels balanced and your weight down.

Finally, your stomach expands and contracts according to the amount of food you load into it, and loses its tone when pushed to the max. So once your stomach is overstretched by large meals in one sitting it takes more food to satisfy you, according to research at St Luke's Roosevelt Hospital in New York. Conversely, eating small meals throughout the day doesn't empty or stretch the stomach so you feel full more quickly.

Take action

- **Never leave more than two or three hours between meals and snacks.** Aim to start the day with breakfast

then have a mid-morning snack, followed by lunch, a
teatime snack and then a light supper.

- **Never skip breakfast.** Breakfast should be your most
important meal because it wakes up your metabolism,
gives you an energy boost and gets you going for the day.
If you don't feel like eating when you get up, try waking
15 minutes earlier or laying the breakfast table the
evening before to motivate you.
- **Eat more of your calories early in the day.** Make sure
you have a good lunch and a light supper so you have a
chance to use up the calories by being active. If you eat a
lot in the evening then go to bed you just confuse your
metabolism and are more likely to put on weight.
- **Eat healthy snacks.** Between breakfast and lunch and
between lunch and supper have a light snack. Make sure
it includes a little protein. You'll find out why later on but
for now the healthy snack suggestions below will get you
thinking along the right lines.

Your Snack Prescription

A healthy snack doesn't mean a couple of chocolate digestives and a milky
coffee. Try these instead:

- Piece of immune-boosting fruit with a few mood-balancing nuts and seeds.
- Slice of fibre-rich wholemeal or rye bread spread with skin-smoothing
almond butter.
- Hormone-balancing hummus spread on a craving-busting oatcake.
- A bone-strengthening low-fat plain yoghurt with some anti-ageing berries.
- Place nutritious and delicious bite-size pieces of seasonal fruit on kebab
skewers and sprinkle with seeds.
- If you crave chocolate try three squares of dark chocolate and three
whole almonds. You'll save on calories and gain heart-healthy
antioxidants and wrinkle-busting essential fats.
- If you crave crisps try wholemeal pitta with spicy salsa instead. You'll
save on calories and gain heart-healthy antioxidants and circulation-
boosting spices.
- If you crave cheese swap for hummus and crudités. You'll save on calories
and gain energy-boosting protein and hormone-balancing phytoestrogens.

Step Three: Say the F-word

Make sure your diet is rich in fibre. Fibre is best known for its beneficial effects on digestion but the amount of fibre in your diet also determines how much oestrogen you excrete and how much you store, making it very important during menopause. Soluble fibre found in fruits, oats and beans binds with toxins so they are excreted. Soluble fibre also binds with some of the cholesterol in the foods we eat, thereby keeping cholesterol levels down and reducing the risk of heart disease.

Fibre is important for weight control too because it slows down the conversion of carbohydrates into sugar. This helps you feel full after you've eaten and reduces the tendency to overeat.

Take action

- **Go for fibre-rich whole foods.** Whole foods are unrefined and in their most natural form. They are naturally bursting with fibre and nutrients to help balance your hormones and boost your metabolism. Whole foods don't contain artificial colourings, flavourings or preservatives. Your body loves whole foods because it gets all that goodness without having to waste energy trying to get rid of all the junk. Fresh vegetables, fruits, wholegrain cereals and breads, legumes (peas and beans), salads, nuts and seeds are all whole foods so eat lots of them.

- **Choose brown rather than white cereals and bread** as they are higher in fibre. Avoid refined flours and bran as they have little nutritional value and act too quickly, preventing you from absorbing nutrients. Healthy flours include wholemeal, quinoa, maize, rye, oat, barley, wheat germ and brown rice. Buckwheat and millet aren't grains but they make good alternatives.

- **Take it slowly.** If you aren't used to a fibre-rich diet, introduce it slowly to give your digestive system time to adjust.

Step Four: Pass on the Sugar

Once you've got used to eating regularly and having more whole foods you're ready for the next stage: monitoring your sugar intake.

Sugar has been linked to numerous health problems including cancer, diabetes and heart disease. It contains no nutrients and goes straight into your bloodstream where it raises blood sugar levels and stimulates the release of insulin. This causes blood sugar levels to plummet so you crave more sugar, giving you a brief high again followed by a big slump. It's a vicious circle that can leave you feeling irritable, tired and moody. Sugar can also overwork your liver and make it unable to process oestrogen effectively. This can cause oestrogen levels to fluctuate, which isn't good news during menopause.

Sugar that isn't used up immediately by your body for energy gets converted into fat, something most women don't want or need. The solution is simple: cut down on your sugar intake.

Take action

- **Cut down on foods with added sugar.** Sweets, biscuits, cakes, pies and other processed foods contain added sugar. If you feel your blood sugar level dipping, don't reach for chocolate or sugary snacks that can drive up your blood sugar levels quickly. Instead, eat something that will give you a steady release of sugar. Refined foods such as white bread, white rice, instant potato and cornflakes can act like sugar in your system because they lack fibre so it's always best to stick with whole grains, fresh fruits and vegetables.
- **Check the label.** Start checking food labels as sugar is a hidden ingredient in many foods, especially processed ones. It has many different names including the following: brown sugar, concentrated fruit juice, corn syrup, dextrose, fructose, glucose, honey, lactose, maltose, molasses, raw

sugar and sucrose. You should also opt for fresh fruit rather than canned. Try low-sugar versions of jams and jellies, and if you take sugar in your tea start cutting down gradually. It's best to avoid sugar substitutes and sweeteners as they have been linked to hormonal problems, weight gain and even cancer. If you really need some sweetness, a pinch of sugar is okay but it's much better to add natural sweeteners like fruit or spices such as cinnamon, cardamom, ginger and nutmeg. You might also want to experiment with the sweet and calorie-free herbal alternative Stevia, which you can get from most health food shops.

- **Don't rely on the GI.** The GI (glycaemic index) is based on good sense if you're approaching menopause. The idea is that eating foods which release their sugar content slowly gives you a sustained release of energy, balancing out your blood sugar to stop you feeling hungry and to protect you against sugar cravings. The trouble is you can't rely on the GI to tell you if a food is healthy or not. For example, a Mars bar or ice cream will have a lower GI score than a baked potato because they release sugar more slowly per 100g but it doesn't take a genius to work out which food is more nutritious. This is because fat slows down the release of sugar from food, so unhealthy high-fat foods are often lower on the GI scale.

  If you are thinking about using the GI you need to consider the GI of the whole meal you are eating. That means you can eat high-GI foods like baked potato as long as you combine them with fibre, healthy fat and protein to slow down the release of sugar. It also helps to think about your portion size. A small portion size of a high-GI food that's packed with nutrients – like raisins, parsnips and carrots – can be extremely good for you. (For those in the know, thinking about the portion size of foods on the GI is called the GL or glycaemic load.) If all this sounds confusing, just use your common sense.

Another quick way to work out the impact of a certain food on your blood sugar levels is to think about how refined it is. If it's highly refined – containing lots of sugar, salt, additives and preservatives – it's going to upset your blood sugar balance and trigger symptoms such as headaches, fatigue, mood swings and weight gain. The less refined it is, the less likely it is to send your blood sugar levels soaring.

- **Persevere.** You may find it extremely hard to cut down on sugar but once you make a start and are eating six healthy meals and snacks a day you'll find that your cravings naturally recede because your blood sugar levels are stable. You may think sugar is your friend when you feel low but believe me it isn't. Pass on the sugar.

If You've Got a Sweet Tooth

- If you're craving sweets your healthiest alternative is to go for fresh or dried fruits such as apricots, apples or pears. Fruit is power-packed with nutrients that can give you a natural energy boost.

- Unsweetened low-fat live yoghurt mixed with fruit (or a spoonful of low-fat jam now and again) is a sweet, creamy, satisfying, nutritious and light alternative.

- Instead of guzzling a fizzy drink loaded with sugar, additives and calories, try a smoothie instead. Smoothies are made from the juice of real fruits. They are scrumptious, sweet and full of goodness.

- Try a bowl of hot oat cereal with a pinch of Stevia or maple syrup on top. It will satisfy your sweet tooth, keep hunger at bay and give you a comfort fix at the same time.

- A small bar of good quality dark chocolate is naturally rich in health-boosting properties. In moderation it can offer chocoholics a healthy, low-fat alternative to high-fat, high-sugar chocolate bars.

(See also the tips on comfort eating in Chapter 6.)

Step Five: Rethink Low Fat

Lots of us have spent years thinking low fat, but low fat is a big no-no if you want to lose weight. True, fat is high in calories but if you're approaching menopause it's crucial for your health, skin and waistline. You just need to make sure you're eating the right kinds of fat, in smallish amounts.

Saturated fats, found in dairy products and red meats, raise your cholesterol and increase your risk of heart disease (which already goes up at menopause), obesity and some cancers. You also need to avoid hydrogenated fats and oils as they can increase your risk of heart disease and diabetes. These can be found in the form of fried, oxidised or trans fats in processed foods, margarines and fast food snacks as well as cakes, sweets and biscuits.

Unsaturated fats, found in olive oil, and essential fatty acids (EFAs) like omega 3 and 6, found in oily fish, nuts and seeds, have a protective effect on your heart and will give you healthy hair and joints, smooth skin and improved brain function. EFAs also help with weight loss because they delay the passage of carbohydrates into your bloodstream, keeping blood sugar levels stable and insulin down. In fact, EFAs are one of the best blood sugar stabilisers around, and as you probably realise by now, stable blood sugar levels mean less likelihood of fatigue, mood swings, heart disease, depression and obesity.

Take action

- **Limit your intake of saturated fats.** Choose low-fat dairy products. Opt for white meat and fish instead of red meat. If you must eat red meat go for lean cuts.
- **Avoid trans fats.** These are harder to avoid than saturated fats because they are hidden in margarines, processed foods and snack foods such as biscuits, cakes and crisps. If you've been upping your intake of whole

foods and fibre and cutting down on sugar and refined carbohydrates you may already have cut down on the trans fats in your diet. Instead of margarine it might be better to go for a small amount of butter.

- **Increase your intake of omega 3 and 6 oils.** You're less likely to be deficient in omega 6 because it's more common in Western diets and found in foods such as leafy green vegetables and soya, olive, sunflower and sesame oils. Omega 3s are less common and found in the oils of cold-water fish, such as mackerel, salmon, herrings and sardines, as well as in hemp seeds, flaxseeds, soya oil, nuts and seeds.

- **Eat oily fish.** Aim to eat oily fish at least twice a week but not more than four times. If you don't eat fish you can eat sea vegetables (seaweeds) and up your intake of hemp and flaxseeds – a great source of omega 3. You might like to try a daily dose of three teaspoons of cold-pressed flaxseed oil or three tablespoons of ground flaxseeds. You can also use hemp and flaxseeds in salad dressings and smoothies.

- **Use only cold-pressed vegetable oils.** Of the readily available vegetable oils only three contain both omega 3 and omega 6: flaxseed, hemp and soya oil, so aim to use these. Other oils such as olive and sunflower do contain omega 6, but not enough omega 3.

- **Go nuts.** Nuts such as walnuts, almonds, pecans, brazil and cashew, and seeds such as pumpkin, sunflower, hemp and sesame are good sources of EFAs so try to eat a handful every day, perhaps as a snack between meals or sprinkled on your salad, soup or cereal. You can also use them in baking.

- **Avoid processed and refined foods.** This is a great way to ensure you get more EFAs in your diet as highly processed foods block their absorption.

Step Six: Give Yourself a Daily Protein Check

A daily protein check is important because protein plays a fundamental role in maintaining your blood sugar balance. If you eat protein with a sugary food it will slow down the conversion of sugar. But this isn't the only reason why protein is important for women over 40. It's also crucial for hormone balance and the metabolism of fat.

Our bodies can't store protein as they can carbohydrate and fat so you need a constant supply. That's why it's important to eat some good quality protein with every meal and snack. Don't go overboard, however, as too much protein leaves less room for all the nutrient-rich carbohydrates and fats we need to balance blood sugar and boost energy. A high-protein diet can also lead to an increased risk of diabetes and heart disease. That's why you need to eat some good quality protein with every meal while making sure you *also* eat nutritious and healthy carbohydrates and fats as part of a varied and balanced diet.

Take action

- **Include a range of low-fat protein in your diet.** Make sure you have a serving with every meal in the form of low-fat cheese, low-fat milk, low-fat yoghurt, lean meat, poultry, seafood, fish, nuts and seeds. Other great sources of protein include soya beans, peas, kidney beans, wheat germ, lima beans, blacked-eyed peas, lentils, black beans, spirulina and grains such as quinoa, wholegrain cereals, soya products, tofu products and Quorn.
- **Eat eggs.** Try to eat at least two or three eggs a week, five if you're a vegetarian. Eggs are a good source of protein and lecithin, a kind of biological detergent that can help break down fat. Lecithin also prevents the accumulation of too many toxic substances in the blood and encourages

the transportation of nutrients through the cell walls. (Eggs should be soft-boiled or poached, since a hard yolk binds the lecithin and limits its detergent action.)

- **Choose skimmed milk.** If you can tolerate dairy products go for skimmed milk rather than the full-fat version. Researchers from the University of Navarra followed the dairy consumption of 6,000 people between 2003 and 2005. They found those who drank skimmed milk and took other dairy products, but not full-fat milk, were 50 per cent less likely to suffer from high blood pressure compared to those who consumed little or no skimmed milk and dairy products.

- **Get the balance right.** Aim to get about 25 per cent of your total daily calories from protein sources, 20 to 25 per cent from healthy fats and the rest from carbohydrates in the form of whole grains, fruit and vegetables.

Protein Sources for Vegetarians and Vegans

There's a popular misconception that meat is the only real source of protein, and thus that a vegetarian diet is inherently unhealthy due to a lack of protein. It's important to stress how untrue this is. There are many protein-rich vegetarian and vegan foods. The only problem is that plant sources of protein, with the exception of soya beans and quinoa, are not complete proteins, so you need to eat more than one in order to get the complete protein.

Vegan sources of protein

- Cereals and grains – wheat, rye, corn, rice, pasta, quinoa
- Leafy green vegetables, including spinach
- Legumes – beans, lentils, peas, peanuts
- Nuts – almonds, walnuts, cashews
- Seaweed – kelp, spirulina
- Seeds – sesame, sunflower
- Soya products – tofu, tempeh, soya milk
- Vegetables – Brussels sprouts, potatoes, yuca

Protein Sources for Vegetarians and Vegans (Cont.)

Vegetarian sources of protein
- Eggs
- Cheese
- Milk
- Yoghurt

If you are the only vegetarian in your house make sure you substitute pulses, beans, wholegrain cereals, dairy products, tofu products or Quorn instead of just omitting the meat part of the meal. Nuts, seeds, grains, pulses and veggies are great sources of protein. Try to eat 30g of nuts and seeds a day and at least four or five soft-boiled eggs a week. To be absolutely certain that you are getting enough protein, you should eat food combinations which form a complete protein, such as:

- Legumes + seeds
- Legumes + nuts
- Legumes + low-fat dairy
- Whole grains + legumes
- Grains + dairy

Chances are you already eat complete proteins without even trying. Here are some tasty and healthy complete protein combinations:

- Beans on wholegrain toast
- Cereal/muesli with skimmed milk
- Granola with yoghurt
- Hummus and pitta bread
- Nut butter with wholegrain bread
- Pasta with low-fat cheese (e.g. lasagne, macaroni cheese)
- Rice and beans, peas or lentils
- Rice with skimmed milk (rice pudding)
- Split pea soup with wholegrain or seeded crackers or bread
- Veggie burgers on wholemeal bread

As well as protein, vegetarian and vegan diets can often be at risk of certain vitamin and mineral deficiencies. To ensure this isn't the case your diet needs to be well balanced. Eat lashings of vegetables and fruit every day and 30g of nuts and seeds. Buy cereals fortified with vitamins, particularly B12. Try to eat a large portion of green leafy vegetables each day, and drink half a pint of skimmed or soya milk to ensure you get your calcium intake. Dried fruits, pulses, green veggies, dark chocolate and whole grains are good sources of iron, and choose butter fortified with vitamin D and E. Taking a good multivitamin and mineral is a sensible idea whether you are vegetarian or a vegan.

Step Seven: Raise Your Glass

Headaches, fatigue, dizziness and bloating are all symptoms of menopause but they can also be symptoms of dehydration. Your body comprises two-thirds water, and you need to drink lots of water to keep your hormonal systems working at their best. Water also keeps your skin healthy and your eyes sparkling. It delivers nutrients to your organs and helps your body eliminate waste and toxins. Finally, water also helps your body metabolise stored fat by maximising muscle function, so it's crucial for weight management.

Take action

- **Drink lots of water.** You need to drink at least six to eight glasses a day, and more if you're exercising or flying. The best source of water is plain, pure drinking water. Water can be contaminated with toxins so if bottled water is too expensive use a water filter for your tap water. If you get bored with plain water, add a bit of lemon or lime for a touch of flavour. Although you can buy flavoured water, some brands contain sugar or artificial sweeteners.
- **Choose other drinks carefully.** Fizzy drinks are best avoided as they tend to contain lots of sugar. Fruit juices are fine but make sure you check the sugar content. Sports drinks contain energy-boosting electrolytes; just look out for added sugar and check the calorie content. Tea and coffee don't really count as sources of water (you'll see why in Chapter 4) so try some herbal tea.
- **Drink fluids at room temperature.** In traditional Chinese medicine, cold drinks disrupt the proper flow of energy and 'shock' the body so stick to fluids that are warm or at room temperature.
- **Take your water with you.** One way to make sure you're drinking enough fluid is to fill a bottle with your

target amount of water and drink it throughout the day. Take it with you in the car or to work and keep it nearby. If the container is empty by bedtime you've achieved your goal.

Step Eight: Spice up Your Life

If you have problems with water retention, bloating and weight gain, this could have nothing to do with the menopause and everything to do with the fact that you have too much salt in your diet.

The more salt you eat, the more your body holds on to water in your tissues to avoid dehydration. A diet high in salt can also increase your risk of high blood pressure. You can't avoid salt altogether but you can take steps to reduce your sodium intake. Have fun experimenting with spices and alternatives until you find those that you like best.

Take action

- **Experiment with other flavourings.** Try using different herbs and spices, wine, lemon juice, vinegar, onions, garlic and chillies instead of automatically adding salt to your food. Take the salt cellar off the table and start cutting down on the amount you use in cooking. In time you'll get used to a less salty diet and start to really taste food again.
- **Check the salt content of foods.** There is salt in most of the foods we buy today, especially those that also contain chemicals, additives and preservatives. Some foods claim to be 'reduced salt' or 'low salt' but this can be misleading. Most manufacturers use the term 'sodium' for salt. To find out how much salt there is in the food you buy, multiply the sodium content by 2.5. Aim for less than 6g of sodium/salt a day.

- **Try a salt substitute.** If you just can't get used to going without salt, try a salt substitute such as LoSalt. Sea salt is richer in natural minerals and lower in sodium than table salt.
- **Avoid salty foods.** These include cured or smoked meats, smoked and pickled fish, tinned meats, salted nuts, salted butter, biscuits, and vegetables in brine. Always go for the low-salt alternative such as fresh fruit, fresh vegetables, fresh lean meat, unsalted butter and nuts, dried fruit, olives in oil and low-salt versions of sauces.

If you've been working through the previous steps of the Menopause Diet, you should find the final two changes very easy as you'll probably be doing them already without realising. The health and weight-loss benefits of these final two recommendations are so potent for women approaching menopause that they deserve special emphasis.

Step Nine: Stock up on Antioxidants

Antioxidants are a group of vitamins, minerals and unique compounds with incredible health benefits for women approaching menopause. They fight the damaging effects of free radicals. These nasty substances are produced by simple bodily functions, such as breathing, and lifestyle habits, such as smoking. They can wreak havoc at a cellular level and make you more susceptible to heart disease, weight gain, cancer and signs of premature ageing (wrinkles).

Our bodies can produce antioxidants naturally, but in the polluted world we live in today we need more antioxidants than our bodies can provide. The best solution is to eat more of them.

Take action

- **Eat antioxidant-rich foods.** Fortunately, antioxidants can be found in many foods. Those rich in vitamins C, E and betacarotene (the plant form of vitamin A) all have antioxidant properties, as do foods rich in the minerals selenium and zinc. Some important plant chemicals are also antioxidants such as lycopene (found in tomatoes), bioflavonoids (found in citrus fruits) and proanthocyanidins (found in berries, grapes and green tea). If you're already eating a whole-food diet with lashings of grains, vegetables and fruit, your antioxidant intake is likely to be just fine. Try to avoid peeling fruits and vegetables as the skin often contains valuable antioxidants.

Antioxidant Power Foods

Vitamin A: Red, orange, deep-yellow and some dark-green leafy vegetables, carrots, sweet potatoes, broccoli, apricots, cantaloupe, mangoes, red and yellow peppers.

Vitamin C: Fruits, especially citrus fruits, green leafy vegetables such as broccoli, berries, sweet peppers and sweet potatoes.

Vitamin E: Cold-pressed vegetable oils, wheat germ, wholegrain products, seeds, nuts and oily fish.

Selenium: Seafood, red meats, poultry, brazil nuts, cereals, barley and other grains and breads.

Zinc: Spinach, broccoli, green peas, green beans, tomato juice, lentils, oysters, prawns, crab, turkey (dark meat), lean ham, lean minced beef, sunflower seeds, oily fish, lean sirloin steak, plain yoghurt, Swiss cheese, almonds, tofu, ricotta cheese.

- **Eat at least five servings of antioxidant fruit and veg a day.** Fruits and vegetables have been found to prevent a host of diseases by providing essential vitamins, minerals, fibre and other nutrients, including antioxidants. If you're not used to eating so many vegetables and fruits a day, this can sound daunting, but it really isn't. One vegetable portion is a mug of raw vegetables or a small cup (8 oz) of cooked veg. A fruit portion is one medium banana, orange or apple. Always eat your fruit with some protein, like some low-fat cheese or a handful of nuts. This is because some fruits, particularly bananas and raisins, can upset your blood sugar levels if eaten alone.

- **Add fruit and veg to your cooking.** If family members aren't used to eating so much fruit and veg, find sneaky ways to add them into your diet and your cooking. For example, you could add sliced apples to the chicken roast, grated carrots and courgette to spaghetti sauce or frozen mixed vegetables to your favourite pasta recipe. You could top ice cream with strawberries or treat everyone to a colourful stir-fry. Try stir-frying peas, pepper strips, bean sprouts and Chinese cabbage, or a mixture of sweetcorn, small chunks of carrot and peas.

- **Choose meals that are packed with veggies.** Craving soup for dinner? Choose a chunky vegetable stew. Pasta on the menu tonight? Remember that tomato-based spaghetti sauce counts as a vegetable. Having pizza for lunch? Buy one with added mushrooms, green peppers and onions; then add your own broccoli when you get home. When cooking and preparing vegetables, cut, slice, dice or shred them into very small pieces. Not only will they 'hide' easily, but small pieces also cook more quickly and blend into your recipe with no trouble.

- **Make snacking fruitful.** Keep baby carrots in a handy spot in the fridge. Place a bowl of seasonal fresh fruit on the counter where it just begs to be eaten. Toss small boxes or plastic bags of dried fruit in your car's glove compartment. When you want a snack, you don't want to wash and peel; you want to eat.

- **Eat your greens.** Cruciferous vegetables, like cabbage, broccoli and Brussels sprouts, deserve special mention here. As well as being potent anti-ageing antioxidants that offer protection against cancer, they also contain a compound called indol-3-carbinol that speeds up the elimination of hormones the body can't use any more so they are less harmful.

- **Drink your produce.** Choose 100 per cent fruit and vegetable juices that are low in sodium. A 12fl oz glass of banana and apple smoothie equals two servings of fruit, so this is an easy and delicious way to add fruit to your diet. Juices, smoothies, soups and frozen vegetables all count towards your daily antioxidant intake.

- **Eat raw.** To maximise their antioxidant power, eat vegetables raw as cooking can destroy nutrients. The next best thing is to steam or stir-fry rather than boil, and if you must boil, boil lightly and keep the nutrient-rich water or stock to use in soups or veggie smoothies.

Exceedingly Good Sources of Antioxidants

Red wine: Two glasses of red wine a day provide a great source of antioxidants. More than this will have the opposite effect and leave you less able to fight off infections. Red wine contains bioflavonoids that help reduce blood clots and therefore strokes.

Dark chocolate: Dark (not milk) chocolate provides one of the richest sources of metabolism-boosting antioxidants called catechins. Although good for you, chocolate in itself is still a fattening food so remember the 80/20 rule (*see page 29*) and eat it in moderation.

Brazil nuts: Brazils are rich in selenium, and as few as three nuts a day will fill your requirements. Cashews, walnuts and almonds are nearly as good. Research has shown that when selenium levels are too low in the body, the risk of cancer is greatly increased.

Blueberries: There is evidence that antioxidant chemicals in blueberries can actually reverse age-related memory loss.

Green tea: Green tea is a far healthier choice than black tea, although all teas are good at reducing the risk of heart disease by boosting the antioxidant action in blood plasma. A single cup of green tea a day brings great health benefits. Studies show that green tea drinkers are 46 per cent less likely to develop hypertension, but watch out for the tannin. Tannin in tea can inhibit vital iron absorption, so don't drink too much. Excessive drinking of black

(Indian) tea (in other words to the degree that the British drink) can cause bladder deficiency through excessive tannin intake. This eventually shows up in old people as incontinence. Two cups of tea a day are sufficient.

Step Ten: Phytoestrogens – Are You Getting Enough?

Phytoestrogens can have a dramatic effect on the symptoms of menopause. Every woman over 40 should ensure she is getting enough.

Phytoestrogens are substances found in certain foods. They have a similar chemical structure to the oestrogen your body produces, and this may explain their hormone-balancing effect. Studies show that they can not only take the place of natural oestrogens and increase oestrogen levels when they are too low, but they can also reduce them when they are too high. As well as helping to balance hormones, phytoestrogens are thought to have a protective effect on the heart. Studies show they can lower levels of bad cholesterol. In addition, they may contain compounds that can inhibit breast and endometrial cancer (often due to excess oestrogen), fibroids and osteoporosis.

Phytoestrogens mainly fall into the class of:

- Isoflavones – the richest source, found in legumes such as lentils and soya beans and chickpeas.
- Lignans – found in nearly all grains and vegetables, the best source being flaxseeds.
- Coumestans – found mainly in alfalfa and mung bean sprouts.

In Japan, where women have as much as one thousand times higher levels of isoflavones in their soya-based diet than the amount found in British and American diets, the average age of menopause is 55 compared to 51 in the West. Breast cancer rates are also much lower and there isn't even a word for 'hot flushes', suggesting that they don't experience them as we do.

There are numerous research papers on the beneficial effects of phytoestrogens and isoflavones on hormone balance at menopause. In a remarkable study reported in the *British Medical Journal*, women going through menopause had their normal diet supplemented with phytoestrogen-rich soya flour and red clover sprouts. This change in diet reduced the amount of FSH (the hormone that rises at menopause) to pre-menopausal levels. The effect of the phytoestrogens was strong enough to reduce vaginal dryness and irritation and ease hot flushes. The study demonstrates that phytoestrogens may be crucial in warding off the symptoms of perimenopause and easing the transition to post-menopause.

Although research has tended to focus on soya, which is a fine source of phytoestrogen, there are plenty of other forms. These include:

- Whole grains such as brown rice
- Oats
- Legumes
- Chickpeas
- Lentils
- Fennel
- Garlic
- Celery
- Parsley
- Hops
- Vegetables, particularly green leafy or cruciferous vegetables such as broccoli, cabbage and Brussels sprouts
- Cinnamon
- Sage
- Red clover
- Seeds: flaxseeds, sesame, pumpkin, poppy, caraway and sunflower

As well as having a beneficial effect on women, it seems that phytoestrogens may also have a protective hormone-balancing effect on men. In Japan, the death rate from prostate cancer is lower than in the West.

Take action

- **Get enough isoflavones.** The recommended amount of isoflavones for women is about 45mg a day. How long it takes before the effects are felt will vary from woman to woman, but is normally around four to eight weeks. It depends on how severe your symptoms are and how healthy you are to start with. Try to eat one serving of soya a day, which is around 55g/2oz. This will give you around 40g of isoflavones. You could also take one tablespoon of flaxseeds a day. Remember, you don't always have to eat soya; other legumes, such as chickpeas and lentils, are good sources of phytoestrogens too.
- **Choose good sources of soya.** There's been some concern about the aluminium levels in soya, which have been linked to Alzheimer's disease. Eaten in moderation, however – say five times a week – soya can reduce cholesterol levels and protect against heart disease. The best way to eat soya is in its traditional form, choosing products such as miso, tofu or organic soya. Avoid snack bars made from whole soya beans.

If you're avoiding processed and refined foods, eating a whole-food diet with plenty of vegetables and fruits and making sure you're getting enough healthy fat and protein, the chances are you're getting enough antioxidants, phytoestrogens and all the other good things you need to help balance your hormones and beat your symptoms.

Seven Golden Rules

1. Eat at least three meals and two snacks a day. Make hunger a thing of the past.

2. Divide your plate: when you sit down for lunch or dinner, draw a couple of imaginary lines to divide your plate into four. About a quarter of your plate should be filled with whole grains; another quarter should be protein. That leaves half of your plate to fill with vegetables, fruit and salad.

3. Cut down on the S-words: sugar, salt and saturated fat, and increase the F-words: fibre, fluids and fish.

4. Eat some quality protein at each meal and snack.

5. Eat a wide variety of fresh fruits and vegetables daily.

6. Eat healthy fats each day.

7. Eat all foods in moderation and enjoy experimenting with new flavours.

The Menopause Diet Detox Boost

Every day we are surrounded by a sea of chemicals that could disrupt our hormones. These are found in everything from solvents, plastics, car fumes and adhesives to substances such as alcohol, cigarettes, make-up and deodorants. Pesticides and herbicides are found in foods, not to mention the additives and preservatives used in processed foods. Even our water contains contaminants.

Substances that mimic our natural hormones are known as HAA (haloaretic acid) chemicals. They include petro-chemicals, xenoestrogens and endocrine-disrupting chemicals (EDCS). Preliminary research shows how potentially damaging the effects of these chemicals can be to our hormonal and general health. Xenoestrogens may increase the risk of early menopause as well as infertility and cancer.

Your body doesn't need or want these toxins and has to work extremely hard to get rid of them. In the process of metabolising these toxins, your body loses vital nutrients – nutrients you need to feel healthy, lose weight and beat the symptoms of menopause.

The answer is to help your body get rid of these unwanted toxins; but don't try to do this by going on a faddy detox diet.

Why Detox Diets are a Waste of Time

In a recent report by the charity Sense About Science, some of the UK's top scientists and toxicologists suggested that faddy detox diets are a waste of time and money.

Eating nothing but cabbage soup or sipping only freshly squeezed ewe's milk for days on end will cause your blood sugar levels to sink really low. This will make you crave stodgy food and leave you feeling extra moody, tired and sluggish. Plus you'll be missing out on essential mood-boosting, fat-burning nutrients like omega 3 fats and protein. It's much better to drink plenty of water, eat cleansing, natural foods and just cut out the bad stuff like saturated fats and sugar. If you've started following the Menopause Diet you should already be eating a diet based on fresh, naturally cleansing foods.

Another reason the average detox diet is a waste of time and money is that your body is constantly detoxifying itself. If anything nasty gets in, your liver will combine it with its own chemicals to make a solution that your kidneys can flush away in your urine or through your skin as sweat. All day, every day, your stomach, liver, kidneys, adrenal glands and lymphatic system work to keep your body free of toxins and you feeling healthy and vital. In fact, these organs are crucial for the removal of the toxins that can clog up your system and make it harder for you to lose weight. The tips that follow will give you a 'no sweat' menopause detox boost.

Step One: Drink Enough Pure Water

The first and biggest menopause detox rule mirrors Step Seven in the Menopause Diet (*see Chapter 3, page 41*). It is to drink more water because water cleanses and helps rehydrate your liver. Don't drink any water you can get your hands on, however; make sure it's pure water.

Your In-house Detox System

Your liver is a chemical clearing house. Every minute of the day it cleans 1.5 litres (3 pints) of blood and neutralises toxic wastes, sending them off to the kidneys and lymph for elimination. It's also your liver's job to convert oestradiol (a more toxic form of oestrogen) into the less toxic oestrone and oestriol, so it's especially important that the liver is working efficiently as you get older. In addition, it produces amino acids and enzymes to metabolise fat, proteins and carbohydrates and helps regulate blood sugar levels. Healthy liver function is therefore crucial not just for detoxification but also for weight loss.

Drugs, alcohol, fatty food, smoking and environmental toxins can overload the liver. If the liver is overloaded it will force your other detoxifying organs (skin, lymph, kidneys, adrenals) to work overtime, which can cause rashes, acne, hormone imbalance, bloating, yeast infections and poor health in general.

To keep your body's detox system in good working order and protect yourself from toxins there are two things you need to do:

1. Give it nutritional support by eating healthily. A healthy diet can help your liver process, transform or eliminate toxins and excess hormones. Follow the Menopause Diet guidelines and make extra sure you get plenty of antioxidants, those protective substances that patrol your body, mopping up toxins (*see Chapter 3, page 43*).
2. Reduce the amount of toxins you're exposed to so that your body's natural detoxification systems can function properly. This Detox Boost is designed to help you do just that. Before you start, don't panic. Just as the Menopause Diet isn't like any other diet, your menopause detox isn't like any other detox. It won't leave you tearful and starving, and you won't hate every minute. You don't need to go on fasts or retreats to detox; all you need to do is avoid unnecessary toxins, and the only side-effect is a feeling of lightness and wellbeing.

It's estimated that as many as 60,000 different chemicals now contaminate our water supply. In addition to man-made oestrogens, a 2004 report found traces of Prozac and seven other drugs in the UK water supply. The standard purification techniques used by most water companies simply don't remove all these chemicals, and they often add more in the form of chlorine and aluminium.

The recognition that much of our tap water is contaminated has led to a boom in bottled water sales. The trouble is, the next bottle of water you drink may be nothing more than tap water that has passed through a filter. There is also little need to drink mineral water. The best way to up your mineral intake is to eat vegetables grown in mineral-rich soil. Distilled water isn't much better as the process of distillation can concentrate some compounds and remove essential trace elements. For water to be pure it must be double distilled, and not many companies do this.

The cheapest and easiest way to ensure the water you're drinking is clean and pure is to purify it in your home with a water filter. Water filter jugs are readily available at supermarkets. Use the filtered water for cooking as well as for hot and cold drinks. Bear in mind that filters can become breeding grounds for bacteria so regularly replace the filter and clean the jug. A good-quality filter should eliminate or greatly reduce the levels of heavy metals such as lead, cadmium and chlorine and remove any adverse tastes, colours and smells in the water. Alternatively, buy water bottled in glass as plastic bottles can increase the amount of toxins in the water. Or drink cooled boiled tap water – this at least gets rid of the bacteria and removes the amount of limescale you're drinking.

Step Two: Eat Fresh

Eat fresh, natural foods whenever possible because they contain the nutrients your body needs to support its in-house detox system. Fresh food also increases your intake of cleansing fibre, which not only encourages elimination but also prevents the absorption of toxins into your bloodstream. If you're eating more fresh food you're less likely to be eating nutrient-scarce ready meals and sugary, fatty, processed and refined foods that bombard your liver with chemicals, additives and lots of dehydrating salt.

There's detox power in fresh food, especially if it's raw or as close to its natural state as possible. Raw food is loaded with nutrients and enzymes. Vital to life, enzymes work tirelessly at breaking down food, assisting the digestive system, boosting the immune system and removing toxins from the body. This isn't to say you should only eat raw food – your digestive system simply couldn't take that – but try to make sure you eat plenty of it. For those who feel they haven't got time to prepare fresh food there are easy ways to incorporate more of them into your life:

- Keep fresh fruit and vegetables handy at all times, even at work.
- Meals could be prepared at weekends and then stored in the freezer for during the week.
- You can order fresh food every few days via the internet, mail order or phone services.
- Soups and salads made from fresh vegetables, grains and legumes are easy to prepare and delicious to eat.
- Tiered steamers can be used to cook fresh fish and vegetables at the same time.
- You can add your own fresh vegetables and toppings to pizza bases.
- Wholemeal bread with chicken, tuna or tofu with a side salad makes for a quick, easy and fresh light meal.

Top detox foods

Asparagus: Lightly boil some asparagus until tender; drizzle with a little olive oil and squeeze over some lemon juice. This makes a fantastic starter packed with an amino acid called asparagine, which along with potassium makes it a diuretic and a cleanser. It helps your kidneys flush out toxins and is great for easing bloating.

Beetroot: This cleansing food contains the antioxidant betacyanin which gives it its vivid colour and revs up your liver's detoxifying process. Beetroot tastes great roasted in olive oil and served in a little balsamic vinegar, but to preserve all its vitamins eat it raw, grated on a salad.

Berries: Blueberries, strawberries, raspberries and blackberries are all full of toxin-fighting antioxidants. Blueberries in particular help strengthen your veins and arteries so you get plenty of essential nutrients and oxygen rushing around your body. Add them to cereals, smoothies or fruit salads.

Broccoli: High in vitamin C, broccoli is known for its cancer-fighting properties. It's also packed with glucosinolates like sulphoraphane, which help your liver to process toxins. Dip florets of raw broccoli into hummus, add to stir-fries or lightly steam and serve with fish. As well as being a good source of detoxifying and cleansing fibre, leafy greens like broccoli and cabbage contain abundant supplies of chlorophyll, one of nature's best cleansers and detoxifiers. Chlorophyll is often taken as a dietary supplement for its ability to combine with gut toxins and remove them from the body. It's also sometimes used as a breath freshener.

Cabbage: Red, white, green or bok choy, cabbages are all great detox foods. High in indole 3 carbinol, they help prevent oestrogen from being absorbed in the body while at the same time encouraging its elimination. They are also packed with antioxidants and sulphur-like substances that protect your liver and help it process chemicals. Shred and use in salads or stir-fries.

Flaxseeds: As well as being a good source of essential fats, flaxseeds contain cleansing fibre. They absorb water and expand in the colon, allowing toxins and mucus to be removed. Some people find that ground flaxseeds in a glass of water are an effective remedy for constipation. If you can't stand the taste, add them to fresh fruit or sprinkle ground seeds over smoothies or salads.

Lemons: The yellow colour of lemons comes from their high antioxidant bioflavonoid content. They are great for supporting liver function and help to wash away toxins. Their high potassium content boosts circulation and acts as a diuretic, encouraging the elimination of waste. Squeeze half a lemon into warm water and drink immediately after rising in the morning, or juice along with grapefruit (another great detox food) for a refreshing smoothie.

Papaya and pineapple: Papaya contains papain, an enzyme that encourages the release of waste products and is very soothing to the stomach and digestive tract. Pineapple is also a mild diuretic. Slice them both together and have for breakfast or dessert. Alternatively, mix with garlic, chillies, spring onions, cucumber, tomatoes, coriander and lime to make a tasty salsa for steamed fish.

Peppers: Peppers are packed with detoxifying antioxidants. The active compound, capsaicin, helps boost circulation and aid digestion. Ensure you eat as many brightly coloured foods as possible so you get a wide range of antioxidants.

Smoothies: Fruit and vegetable juices are the cleansers, energisers, builders and regenerators of the human system. A combination of either fresh raw fruit or vegetable juices will supply enzymes, vitamins and minerals to aid the body's natural detoxification and increase vitality. Chop up your favourite fruits or vegetables and place in a blender for a delicious breakfast smoothie or afternoon pick-me-up.

Watercress: Another great source of glucosinolates which help stimulate the liver's detox enzymes. It's also packed with magnesium and calcium so it's a good bone booster. Whip up some watercress soup or use as an alternative to lettuce.

Herbal Helpers

- Herbal teas can boost liver function and help you gently detox. Try alfalfa, burdock, chamomile, dandelion, lemon, red clover, rosehip, nettle and green tea. Sip some throughout the day. Milk thistle is an excellent herb for the liver. Many studies have shown it can increase the number of new liver cells to replace old, damaged ones.

- Castor oil, applied externally, can be used to stimulate the liver and draw out toxins from the body. Apply slightly warmed oil to your stomach with a flannel and leave for one hour.

- Beneficial herbs and spices for the kidneys include goldenrod, cinnamon, cloves, nettle and parsley. Numerous herbs support adrenal function but the most notable are the ginsengs, which should be prescribed by a qualified practitioner.

- Your lymph nodes process and eliminate toxins via the skin so stimulate your lymphatic system with some essential oil massage. Add six drops of ginger and rosemary, five drops of lemon grass and four drops of peppermint essential oil to 30ml base oil and massage over your abdomen.

Step Three: Cook Light

Fresh food can become unhealthy if it's cooked unhealthily. Cooking generally causes nutrient loss which compromises the immune system and leads to fatigue and weight gain. The more a food is cooked – especially vegetables – the higher its sugar content. Proteins, too, aren't spared by cooking. When protein is overcooked the protein itself is destroyed, rendering it at best useless and at worst harmful.

This doesn't mean you shouldn't cook food at all. Certain foods – such as eggs, meat and fish – can be extremely dangerous to eat when raw and need to be cooked thoroughly.

Try to balance cooked food with more raw food, perhaps 50:50, and make sure you follow these healthy cooking tips:

- Cook with olive oil or sunflower oil.
- Include as many raw fruits and vegetables and fresh ingredients as possible in your cooking and avoid processed ones.
- Cook gently and at a lower heat, for longer if necessary, letting your food simmer or steam lightly. When cooking fruits and vegetables it's best to warm them rather than cook them vigorously. A good trick when making soup is to heat the soup and at the last minute add some raw vegetables so that they are just warmed by the soup broth.
- Steaming is the best way to cook vegetables. Stir-frying is good for fish, meat and vegetables. Poaching is useful for eggs and fish. Meat should be roasted since other methods, such as frying, use too much fat.
- Boiling vegetables means losing nutrients into the cooking liquid. If you do boil vegetables keep the water to add to soups and casseroles. (Please note: some ingredients such as dried beans and pulses need to be boiled in plenty of unsalted water until fully cooked.)
- Avoid dishes that require creamy, rich sauces and salt. Use herbs and spices instead.
- As for microwaving, we don't know what molecular changes may be happening to the food when cooked, so it's best to limit its use as much as you can.
- Avoid all aluminium cookware as this is a heavy toxic metal that can enter food through the cooking process. The same applies to wrapping food in aluminium foil. The best cookware to use is cast iron, enamel, glass or stainless steel.

Step Four: Ditch the Bad Fats

A diet high in saturated fats can stimulate oestrogen production and clog up your liver so it can't detox efficiently. You need to ensure you get your essential fats but avoid saturated fats found in meat, dairy products, pies, cakes and biscuits.

You can cut down on meat and dairy products by substituting them with fish or vegetable proteins, such as nuts, pulses and grains. If you eat a lot of meat, try to avoid red meat, such as beef and pork, and go for lean meat instead, such as chicken and turkey. Always cut off the fat.

Cook with oils such as sunflower or olive rather than butter or lard. Try mashed avocado on grainy bread instead of margarine on white; cottage cheese instead of Cheddar; and oils like hemp for salads or dressings.

Full-fat milk products, butter and hard cheese are high in saturated fat and cholesterol so make an exception to the 'Rethink Low Fat' rule in the Menopause Diet (*see Chapter 3, page 36*) and choose low-fat or skimmed milk, yoghurts and cheeses. Milk substitutes such as rice, soya, oat or nut milks are also a good idea. When you buy dairy products, try to buy organic to reduce your intake of chemicals and hormones.

Step Five: If You Smoke, Quit

Smoking damages almost all aspects of your hormonal, sexual and reproductive health. It's a significant anti-nutrient and reduces levels of the antioxidant vitamin C in your bloodstream. Smokers also have high levels of cadmium, a heavy toxic metal that can stop zinc doing its job properly (zinc is needed for healthy hormone function). What's more, smoking drains oestrogen levels. This can increase the risk of early menopause and conditions linked to lower oestrogen levels, such as osteoporosis, regardless of whether you smoke five or 20 cigarettes a day. Other studies link smoking with an increased risk of heart disease, infertility and breast and lung cancer.

Passive smoking, too, has its risks. Just 30 minutes in the company of smokers can damage your heart by reducing its ability to pump blood, according to research published in the *Journal of the American Medical Association* (January, 1998).

In short, smoking leaches nutrients you need to support your health and balance your hormones, so if you're approaching menopause you are strongly advised to quit. Quitting, though, isn't always easy, especially if you've been a smoker for many years. Here are some helpful tips:

- Researchers at the University of Pittsburgh School of Medicine found that women who quit smoking between the first and 14th day of their menstrual cycle had fewer withdrawal symptoms such as depression, anxiety and irritability.
- Your liver and lungs can recover if you stop smoking and support them with the nutrients they need to thrive. The nutritional strategy for smokers is to increase their intake of whole grains, raw seeds, nuts, legumes and fruits and vegetables, and decrease their intake of fats, food additives and alcohol. Since smoking generates an acidic condition in the body, a wholemeal, high-fibre diet helps detoxification by maintaining healthy bowel function. Research at St George's Hospital Medical School, London, published in the medical journal *Thorax* (January, 2000), found that certain foods, such as apples, can boost lung health and healing. Organic, unfiltered, raw apple cider vinegar is a natural tonic for overall health, especially respiratory health. Dilute with water and drink a glass every day.
- Drink lots of water as it's essential to balance out the drying effects of smoking.

- Get counselling. Aim for four to seven sessions over a two-month period with a counsellor who is used to treating addictive conditions. Some people find alternative therapies like acupuncture and hypnotherapy helpful.
- A general multivitamin with additional antioxidant nutrients – vitamins A, C, E, zinc and selenium – is an important part of any smoker's quitting programme. The cadmium won't leave your body when you stop smoking; it needs to be tackled by supplementing your diet with antioxidants.
- Nicotine gums and patches may offer relief.
- Many people say that gradually reducing the amount of cigarettes they smoke a day isn't helpful. You may find that the best way is to go cold turkey and smoke your last cigarette. The nicotine will pass out of your system after 48 hours so you won't be craving it. What you'll be craving is the habit of smoking: using it as a time to relax or to have something to do with your hands. You need to replace smoking with a more positive habit. If you feel like you want a cigarette, go for a walk for your time out. If you don't know what to do with your hands, buy some worry beads. If you crave a smoke after a meal, pop some chewing gum into your mouth.

Step Six: Cut Down on Caffeine and Alcohol

Caffeine and alcohol in moderation are fine; just don't go overboard.

Caffeine

Whether you're drinking coffee, tea or caffeinated soft drinks, low doses of caffeine can make you feel more energetic and alert because caffeine triggers the release of cortisol and other stress hormones. If, however, you drink too much, excess cortisol is released into your bloodstream and this can weaken your adrenals, deplete your body of vital nutrients and interfere with hormonal balance. A cycle develops where ever greater amounts are needed to achieve the familiar high, and symptoms such as headaches, fatigue and indigestion can occur if you don't get your fix. In short, you get addicted. This doesn't mean you need to give up caffeine altogether; it just means you should keep an eye on the amount you're drinking.

In general, studies show that drinking around two or even three cups of tea or coffee a day won't damage your health. It may even give it a boost because tea contains substances called catechins that are thought to protect against heart disease, and coffee contains substances that may help boost memory function in old age and even prevent diabetes. It's the excesses that are dangerous. So if you're drinking more than three cups of tea, coffee or caffeinated drinks a day, you need to cut down.

Your Caffeine Cut-back Plan

■ Make one cup at a time instead of a whole pot and buy a smaller pot so you aren't tempted to drink more.

■ If you're at a coffee shop order a small cup.

■ To ease withdrawal symptoms cut back gradually over two to three weeks. Lower your intake by drinking grain coffee blends, herbal coffees or diluted or smaller amounts of regular coffee.

■ Start cutting back during the weekend or on holiday when you're less busy and stressed. If you get withdrawal symptoms take lots of exercise and warm baths and drink lots of water.

■ Decaffeinated options for tea and coffee aren't really a good choice as we have no idea how many chemicals are involved in the decaffeination process.

■ Experiment with herbal teas such as chamomile, barley, chicory, dandelion, lemon grass, peppermint, ginger root, red clover, rosehip, apple, hibiscus, clover flower and nettle.

Alcohol

Like caffeine, alcohol has both negative and positive effects for women approaching menopause. Let's start with the negative:

- Alcohol interferes with hormonal balance.
- Alcohol is high in calories and can stop you absorbing zinc, which is crucial for hormonal health.
- Alcoholic drinks are often high in sugar and enter your bloodstream very quickly, causing rapid fluctuations in blood sugar balance.
- The liver metabolises alcohol, either converting it to energy or storing it as fat. When too much is consumed, this can interfere with the liver's normal functioning and make it less able to clear out excess hormones and toxins.
- Fat builds up in the liver. Since alcohol converts to fat, obesity is common among those who drink in excess.
- Chronic heavy drinking can increase the risk of breast cancer, weaken bones, cause fertility problems and birth defects and interfere with blood sugar control.

Now let's take a look at the positive effects:

- A small amount of alcohol may be beneficial. It's thought that one or two glasses of red wine a day may decrease the risk of heart disease. This is because red wine contains cardio-protective bioflavonoids.
- Beer and spirits may have the same immune-boosting benefits as red wine.
- Drinking alcohol in small amounts regularly could mean you are less likely to become obese than if you don't drink at all, according to a US study published in the journal *BMC Public Health* (December, 2005).

It's important to stress that research focusing on the positive effects of alcohol is always based on a moderate to low intake. For example, in the BMC study the researchers said the results didn't mean teetotallers should turn to the bottle in the battle of the bulge. In fact, the study indicated that the odds of being overweight or obese were significantly higher among those who indulged in binge drinking and/or heavy drinking, consuming four or more drinks per day. In contrast, light to moderate drinking – consuming one or two drinks per day – was associated with lower odds of being overweight or obese. No more than one or two drinks a day is considered ideal, so if you're drinking more than that you need to cut down.

Step Seven: Protect Yourself from Pesticides and Plastics

Pesticides are chemicals sprayed on crops to protect them from bugs, rodents and bacteria and to make them grow faster. They can also be found in some plastics, herbicides, household products and industrial chemicals. It's estimated that around 359 different pesticides are used on food, on pets or in homes.

Go organic

As we've seen, pesticides contain xenoestrogens, oestrogen-like chemicals that can interfere with the natural process of your hormones (*see page 51*). To reduce your intake, try to buy organic produce as much as possible. Organic foods are generally free of chemicals, growth hormones and antibiotics, and contain higher amounts of vitamins and minerals because they're grown in nutrient-rich soil.

You can find organic produce in most supermarkets these days. If you think organic produce is too expensive, consider buying just one item a week – such as organic brown rice or organic apples – to get you into the habit of looking at it as an investment for your health. Specifically, look for organically grown spinach, peaches, peppers, strawberries, cherries, celery, apples, apricots, green beans, grapes and cucumbers as these foods consistently contain the most pesticides. You could also get mail-order boxes delivered to your door via a local farmer or the internet.

If you eat meat you may want to consider switching to organic produce. For many years cattle, chickens and even farmed fish have been routinely treated with hormones and antibiotics to keep them healthy and to step up their weight gain. More research is needed but a growing number of experts believe these hormones may be adversely affecting our hormonal health and increasing the risk of cancer. Organic meat is produced without the routine use of drugs common in intensive livestock farming.

If your fruits and vegetables are not organic, make sure you rinse them (don't soak them). Washing can't completely remove the chemicals that have been absorbed but it can take away the residue. Remove and discard the outer leaves of cabbages and other greens. Peel fruits and vegetables before using them. If you buy organic you only need to scrub the skins. Eat a wide variety of fruits and vegetables as specific pesticides are used for specific crops and you'll avoid eating too much of a given pesticide.

Be aware of packaging

Tin cans and plastic bottles also contain xenoestrogens so try to reduce your exposure to them. Preliminary research on animals has raised questions about the safety of clingfilm made from PVC, suggesting it may interfere with hormonal health. Until we know more, avoid food and drinks in plastic containers or wrapped in plastics, especially fatty foods because xenoestrogens are fat-loving. If you do buy food in a plastic container, remove it from its packaging as soon as possible. Don't heat – and especially don't microwave – food in plastic, and store food in a glass dish rather than clingfilm. It might also be a good idea to use glass bottles instead of plastic or cans to avoid the small amount of residue that dissolves into drinks from the container.

Step Eight: Read Food Labels

Additives in food include colourings, preservatives, flavour enhancers, emulsifiers and thickeners. These have been linked to a range of health problems including headaches, asthma, allergies, hyperactivity in children and even cancer, and should be avoided, where possible. They can make your body's own detox system less efficient, add to your toxic load and increase the likelihood of irregular periods, acne, hair loss, weight gain and fatigue.

We are fortunate today in that food manufacturers are required to list the ingredients in their products. Despite this, however, studies show that food labels can still be confusing and misleading for consumers. The following guidelines should make things easier for you.

Colourings

A dangerous class of additives, and one of the easiest to avoid, are the dyes capable of interacting with and damaging your immune system, speeding up ageing and even causing cancer. Watch out for labels with any of the following:

- artificial colour added
- the words 'green', 'blue' or 'yellow' followed by a number
- tartrazine (E102)

- quinoline yellow (E104)
- sunset yellow (E110)
- beetroot red (E162)
- caramel (E150) or FD
- C red no 3

Steer clear of artificial colourings. You wouldn't add dyes to the food you cook at home, so why eat them in the foods you buy? Some foods contain natural colours obtained from plants, and these are safe. The most common is annatto, from the reddish seed of a tropical tree. Annatto is often added to cheese to make it more orange or butter to make it more yellow. Also acceptable are red pigments obtained from beets, green from chlorella and carotene from carrots.

Preservatives and other additives

Preservatives extend a food's shelf life. Citric acid and ascorbic acid (vitamin C, ascorbates, E300–4) are safe, natural antioxidants added to a number of foods. However, synthetic additives such as BHA and BHT (E320–21) may not be safe. Other substances to avoid include:

- **Alum:** an aluminium compound used in many brands of pickles to increase crispiness and also found in some antacids and baking powder. Aluminium has no place in human nutrition and you should avoid ingesting it.
- **Nitrates (Nitrites, E249–52):** a type of preservative added to processed meats, such as hot dogs, bacon and ham. Nitrates can create highly carcinogenic substances called nitrosamines in the body. It's best to avoid any products containing sodium nitrate or other nitrates.
- **Monosodium glutamate (MSG or 621):** a natural product long used in East Asian cooking and added to

many manufactured foods as a flavour enhancer. It's an unnecessary source of additional sodium in the diet and can cause allergic reactions. Omit MSG from recipes, don't buy products containing it and when eating Chinese, request that food be made without it.

Other flavour enhancers and preservatives to avoid include monopotassium glutamate (622) and sodium osinate (631), and benzoic acid and benzoates (E210–9) found in soft drinks, beer and salad creams.

Emulsifiers, stabilisers and thickeners are found in sauces, soups, breads, biscuits, cakes, frozen desserts, ice cream, margarine and other spreads, jams, chocolate and milk shakes. They include guar gum (E412), gum Arabic (E414), pectins (E440), cellulose (E460) and glycerol (E422).

As consumers become more health-conscious, we're increasingly seeing food labels proclaiming 'no hidden colouring', 'no artificial sweeteners' or 'no artificial ingredients'. This is helpful, but you still need to watch out for hidden fats, salts and sugars and alternative names for foods that aren't very good for you when eaten in excess. Sugar, for example, has lots of different names, including sucrose, fructose, dextrose, corn syrup, malt syrup and maple syrup. Sodium is just another name for salt. Animal fat is saturated fat, and trans fatty acid is another name for hydrogenated fat. Mannitol, sorbitol, xylitol, saccharine and aspartame are just alternative names for potentially carcinogenic artificial sweeteners.

Some chemicals are harmless, such as ammonium bicarbonate, malic acid, fumaric acid, lactic acid, lecithin, xanathan, calcium chloride, monocalcium phosphate and monopotassium phosphate. But how can you tell when there's a long list of chemical names that look unfamiliar to you? A good general rule is simply to avoid products whose chemical ingredients outnumber the familiar ones.

Step Nine: Chemical-free Living

Since there's a clear link between environmental toxins and hormonal health it makes sense to avoid possible sources of contamination. The following tips for chemical-free living, combined with the advice in the rest of this chapter, will help you do just that:

- **Lose weight.** For some reason, xenoestrogens love fat. They are stored in body fat and overweight people tend to have higher concentrations. Some experts believe that losing weight will help.
- **Get active.** A great detoxifier, exercise boosts circulation, speeds up metabolism, aids digestion, encourages sweating and elimination and clears the mind.
- **Manage stress.** Stress channels your body's energy reserves away from the detoxification systems, so signs of toxicity can worsen if you're having a stressful time. Check out the stress management tips in Step Ten, below.
- **Check chemicals at work.** Carbon disulphide used in several chemical manufacturing processes such as the production of plastics has been linked to hormonal imbalance. Many pesticides and herbicides are known reproductive toxins. People working in gardens, parks, plant nurseries and farms are at risk. Exposure to heavy metals (traffic fumes), solvents (dry-cleaning) and to glycol ethers (used by electronics manufacturing firms) has been linked to fertility problems.
- **Avoid mercury fillings.** Refuse and, when possible, consult a good dentist to replace mercury dental fillings with non-toxic ones. There are also high levels of mercury in tuna fish so keep your intake down to three or four portions a week.
- **Limit electromagnetic radiation.** Devices that emit electromagnetic radiation such as computer monitors, mobile phones and microwaves should be used with

caution and as far away from the bedroom as possible. Preliminary research suggests they could have negative effects on health. Buy battery-operated clocks and radios and unplug electrical sockets before you go to bed. Limit your time spent at computer screens as some research suggests it can increase the risk of eye strain. Take regular breaks, around five minutes every half an hour, and switch the monitor off rather than using the screensaver. An ioniser on top of your desk may help.

- **Choose paints carefully.** Many household paints give off dangerous fumes as they dry. Water-based paints are better because they contain fewer volatile organic compounds (VOCs).

- **Check toys.** Toys made from PVC plastic can contain softeners called phthalates which are suspected hormone disrupters. Ask for PVC-free toys in the shop. (By law, new teething toys for babies should now be free from phthalates.)

- **Check toiletries and cosmetics.** Be especially wary of the aluminium in deodorants as scientists are currently investigating links between deodorants and breast cancer. Use natural cosmetic products and deodorants instead. Most firms keep their ingredients secret, writing 'parfum' on the label. Why not cut down on one or two scented products? Treat your pets or your house with natural herbal sprays. Better still, open a window instead of spraying air-freshener.

- **Check skincare products.** The same goes for skincare and make-up products as they can contain chemicals that are absorbed into the bloodstream. Explore your local health food store or reputable on-line health sites and see what natural alternatives are out there. Tampons – especially super-absorbent ones – may dry the vagina, making the transfer of toxins easier. It's best to use towels instead, but if you do use tampons make sure you change them every four hours. Some studies have found that 100 per cent cotton tampons don't produce toxins.

- **Minimise the chemicals you use in your home.** These include polish, bleach, detergents and air-fresheners. Try to buy natural products or use tried-and-tested cleaners like white vinegar and lemon for stain removal, chemical-free liquid soaps and detergents. Lemon juice is a natural bleach perfect for stubborn stains or wooden chopping boards. If limescale is your bugbear, vinegar is ideal for sinks, baths and taps. Bicarbonate of soda mixed with water dissolves dirt and grease. Used dry, it can help lift carpet stains, and as a powder nothing is better for neutralising odours. For grimy windows mix vinegar with water in a spray bottle and spritz it on. The soft inside of a banana skin is great for wiping dust from indoor plants.

- **Take a walk.** At least once a day try to take a stroll in a park or green place. Trees give out energising oxygen. It's also a good idea to have plants in your home and workplace. NASA research has shown that the following plants can extract fumes, chemicals and smoke from the air: peace lilies, dwarf banana plants, spider plants, weeping figs, geraniums and chrysanthemums.

Taking measures to avoid toxins in your food and the environment can reduce your toxic load. This doesn't mean you can never drink a glass of unfiltered water again or eat a non-organic banana. Remember the 80/20 rule (*see Chapter 3, page 29*): it applies just as much to detoxifying as it does to your diet. If you get it right most of the time you're doing great. You still have to live in the real world, and there's bound to be the odd day when you slip up. Just as you are doing with your eating plan, find a balanced, achievable approach and don't go overboard.

Step Ten: Take it Easy

Finding ways to cope with the stresses and strains of modern life is an essential part of the Menopause Diet Detox Boost. A certain amount of stress is fine, as it reminds us that we are alive, but too much stress can have a toxic effect on your hormones and your health.

When you're stressed your adrenal glands prompt the release of stress hormones such as cortisol into your bloodstream, triggering what's known as the fight or flight response. But instead of fighting or running away, most of us continue fuming at the children/partner/computer/car ahead, and the cortisol and sugar stay in our system, triggering hormone imbalance and weight gain. If you're under long-term stress, your adrenal glands start to wear down and have difficulty producing hormones in the right amount. This can drive your body towards insulin imbalance, hormone imbalance, depression and loss of libido.

Research has also shown that stress-induced cortisol and blood sugar imbalances can trigger weight gain, especially around the middle and abdominal fat is a predictor of heart disease (*see page 19*). Studies show that women with belly fat, whether overweight or not, produce more cortisol than women without belly fat. Women with high levels of cortisol are also more likely to overeat than women without these high levels. So any woman watching her weight at menopause needs to keep a careful eye on her stress levels.

In the long term it's vital for your weight, health and wellbeing that you keep your adrenal glands healthy and don't overuse your stress hormones. The first step in boosting the health of your adrenals is to follow the Menopause Diet guidelines (*see Chapter 3*). This will give your body the tools it needs to perform optimally. Diet is the foundation of good health and can't be overestimated in relation to stress.

Certain nutrients such as the B vitamins – especially B5 and B6, vitamin C and the essential fatty acids can be extremely helpful if stress is a problem, and they will help boost the functioning of your adrenal glands. When stressed, you lose more vitamin C, and this vitamin is vital for keeping the immune system strong. You should be getting these nutrients from your healthy Menopause Diet, but if you're under stress you might want to add more:

- B vitamins, found in nuts and whole grains
- essential fats, found in oily fish, nuts and seeds
- vitamin C, found in citrus fruits

To prevent your adrenals from burning out you also need to be able to distinguish between what's a real stress or emergency and what isn't. Many of the things we get worked up about aren't really that important so it might help to have a rethink about what drives you mad. Changing your attitude and identifying stress triggers can be extremely helpful, but if you still find it hard to cope with stress it's important to be able to deal with it.

Regular exercise is a great stress-buster. Studies show it can reduce the impact of stress, relax the body and boost mood. Deep-breathing exercises, meditation, yoga, t'ai chi and massage are other ways to calm your body and mind. Below you'll find some tried-and-tested stress-busting techniques to use when you feel overwhelmed. Playing a musical instrument, dancing, writing in your diary, watching a funny DVD or anything that specifically helps you relax and unwind are also highly recommended.

Instant stress-busters

- **Take a deep breath.** Close your eyes and take a deep breath. Visualise yourself in peaceful, tranquil surroundings such as on a beach. Focus on something soothing in your environment. You may choose a flower, a colour or anything that soothes you.

- **Concentrate on your breathing**. Slow it down to a 10-second cycle, six breaths a minute. Inhale for five seconds then exhale for five seconds. Do this for about two to five minutes. If this doesn't work, jog on the spot, punch something like a cushion or count to 10.
- **Talk to friends, family or partners.** If you don't feel you can talk to anyone you know, a trained counsellor may help you get in touch with your feelings and give you tips on how to deal with stress.
- **Try a herbal remedy.** Valerian is a sedative that's been shown to help people fall asleep faster and sleep better and longer without causing loss of concentration. Or drink some kombucha tea which contains stress-busting B vitamins and other micronutrients, and is made from a yeast culture.
- **Take time out.** For five minutes every hour, try to 'shut down' and think of nothing but your perfect situation. This could be a dream holiday, ideal partner or simply thinking about doing nothing at all. You'll be surprised at how effectively this can lower stress levels. Daydreaming is a natural stress-busting technique.
- **Try aromatherapy.** Certain aromas are thought to activate the production of the brain's feel-good chemical, serotonin. Add a few drops of one of the following essential oils to a tissue to sniff when you feel stress levels rising: jasmine, neroli, lavender, chamomile, ylang ylang, vetiver, clary sage, lemon, peppermint. You may also want to use essential oils in your bath to help you unwind. When you feel tense, try one of the following: three drops patchouli and three drops of sandalwood; three drops of rosewood and three drops of clary sage; two drops of vetiver and jasmine. If you prefer you could also burn these oils in a vaporiser to help clarify and invigorate your mind.

- **De-clutter.** Mess creates confusion and a sense of loss of power. If your desk, home or car is messy and disorganised, have a good clearout and tidy up. You'll instantly feel more in control.
- **Do a walking meditation.** Simply go for a walk to clear your mind of stress. Focus on your body and its every movement, and breathe in deeply to let go of tension. If your mind wanders, focus on the feeling of your feet moving heel to toe as you walk.
- **Get some music therapy.** Take 10 minutes to listen, dance or sing along to your favourite piece of music each day and you'll be amazed at how much more relaxed you feel. Just make sure you choose something uplifting.
- **Release the tension.** Do you hunch your shoulders when stressed? Do you tighten your fists, cross your arms or wrap your legs around each other? Become aware of the way your body reacts when you're under stress. Then, when you feel yourself going into that stress position, do the opposite – release your shoulders, stretch out your hands, uncross your arms or legs, and don't forget to breathe. Stop frowning: relax your jaw by gently resting the tip of your tongue for a second behind your top front teeth. At the same time, try to consciously relax the facial muscles and let the shoulders drop down and away from your ears by an inch or two – you'll be astonished by how much tension you were holding in your body.

Ayurvedic Stress-buster

Try this Ayurvedic technique for soothing the brain. For as long as possible, gently massage the point above your nose in the middle of the forehead in a very light circular movement. Pressing the loose skin between your thumb and forefinger is also good for reducing stress and convenient when you're on the phone.

- **Drink chamomile tea.** Chamomile is one of the best herbs for relieving tension as it has a gentle sedative effect. Drink a cup any time you feel tense to help you relax. A cup before you go to bed can help you sleep.
- **Get a good night's sleep.** Women approaching menopause often experience disrupted sleep caused by hormonal fluctuations, and when you're tired it's harder to deal with stress. Lack of sleep can also be a trigger for weight gain. For advice and tips on getting a good night's sleep see Chapter 8.
- **Stroke your pet.** If you have a pet, stroke it. It's been proven to lower blood pressure and stress levels. If you haven't got a pet, why not give someone you love a hug? It will have the same effect.
- **Write it down.** When it all seems too much, grab a pen and paper and write down what you need to do. Listing things on paper will also help focus your mind, enabling you to think clearly about what is a priority, what can wait and what can be delegated to someone else. Once a job has been dealt with, be sure to cross it off the list. It's satisfying and stress-busting to watch your list shrink!

Living with the Menopause Diet

Now that you know what to eat and what not to eat at menopause to ease your symptoms and encourage weight loss, here are some ideas to help you plan meals. Experiment with a few of the recipes and then start creating your own. Some menu ideas to get you started are listed below.

First Thing in the Morning

A cup of hot water with some freshly squeezed lemon juice (to hydrate your body, boost your metabolism, balance your blood sugars and boost your intake of antioxidant anti-ageing vitamin C).

Breakfast

Choose from one of the following:

- Fruit smoothie made with mixed berries, soya milk or yoghurt and 1 tbsp mixed seeds or ground flaxseeds /linseeds.
- Two boiled eggs, a slice of wholegrain toast and a glass of freshly made apple and carrot juice.
- Oat porridge sprinkled with nuts and seeds – such as almonds, flaxseeds/linseeds and sunflower seeds – and a chopped pear with a cup of tea.

- Wholegrain cereal, skimmed milk and berries with a glass of homemade apple, pear and berry juice (*see recipe on page 82*).
- Poached egg on a slice of wholegrain toast with a grilled tomato and a glass of apple juice.

Breakfast Smoothies

Banana and pineapple smoothie. You will need 1 banana, 2 spears of pineapple and 3 tbsp low-fat yoghurt. Peel the banana and break into chunks. Remove the pineapple skin and cut into spears then chunks. Blend the yoghurt, banana and pineapple until smooth.

Banana and peach smoothie with berries. You will need 1 banana, 2 peaches, 12 strawberries, raspberries or blueberries and 3 tbsp low-fat yoghurt. Peel and cut the banana. Peel and remove the stones from the peaches and cut into chunks. Wash the berries and remove any stalks. Blend all the ingredients until smooth.

Lunch

Enjoy one of the following:

- Homemade watercress soup served with 2 slices of wholemeal bread.
- Baked potato topped with ratatouille and hummus.
- Wholemeal pitta bread with tuna or cottage cheese and salad. Piece of fresh fruit.
- Grilled chicken with large mixed salad, half a chopped avocado, lemon and olive oil dressing with a small wholegrain roll.
- Mixed bean salad with tomatoes, half an avocado, walnuts, cucumbers, peppers and olive oil and balsamic vinegar dressing.
- Homemade mixed vegetable and cannellini bean soup, wholegrain roll with cottage cheese.

- Large mixed salad including beetroot, watercress, peppers and tomatoes. Toss in olive oil and lemon juice, season and sprinkle over some nuts and seeds for protein or add half a tin of tuna in spring water.
- Homemade tomato, pepper and onion soup with mixed salad on wholemeal toast.

Dinner
Sample one of the following:

- Lightly grilled tuna served with a small portion of brown rice and stir-fried mixed vegetables including shredded cabbage, broccoli, peppers, spring onions and carrots. Dessert: a fruit salad made with your favourite fruits, such as mango, banana, berries, apple or pineapple. Cut into bite-size chunks and toss with some fresh mint leaves.
- Baked salmon and a large mixed salad sprinkled with nuts and seeds, dressed with lemon and olive oil. Dessert: fruit compote with low-fat natural yoghurt.
- Grilled fish served with lightly steamed asparagus drizzled with olive oil and lemon juice, and a mixed salad. Dessert: homemade berry compote with 1 tbsp fat-free natural yoghurt.
- Chicken and vegetable stir-fry with ginger, garlic and brown rice. Dessert: oaty fruit crumble with a small scoop of ice cream.
- Homemade mince or Quorn bolognaise with plenty of vegetables (courgettes, peppers, celery and aubergines) with wholemeal pasta and salad. Dessert: grilled fruit.
- Stir-fried rice noodles plus grilled chicken breast with fresh pineapple and coriander salsa, and stir-fried vegetables such as broccoli, mangetout and baby sweetcorn. Dessert: frozen berries with low-fat yoghurt and a drizzle of honey.

- Grilled chicken or marinated tofu kebabs with brown rice, roasted Mediterranean vegetables and hummus. Dessert: baked apple with low-fat natural yoghurt.

Nutrient-packed Snacks

- Couple of squares of dark chocolate (70 per cent cocoa solids) so you get plenty of antioxidants and calcium.
- A small piece of fruit with a handful of nuts and seeds for your antioxidants, fibre and essential fats.
- 2 tbsp hummus and crudités for antioxidants and phytoestrogens.
- Low-fat natural yoghurt with nuts and seeds for protein, calcium and essential fats.
- Oat cake and half a mashed avocado for essential fats, antioxidants and slow-release carbohydrates.
- Cup of herbal tea and digestive biscuit.
- Wholemeal pitta bread, scraping of low-fat mayo and fresh vegetable crudités such as carrots sticks, strips of red and yellow pepper and raw broccoli florets.
- Apple, pear and berry juice. You will need 2 apples, 1 pear and about a dozen berries. Keep a few pieces of apple to put through the juicer last to help flush the thicker berry juice through the machine. Apples and pears taste sublime when juiced together. Berries are packed with nutrients, especially potassium, and any berry – strawberry, raspberry, blackberry – works well with apple and pear.
- Tofu shake. You will need 115g/4oz tofu, 1 cup/8oz of fresh or frozen fruit (according to taste), ½ cup/4oz of water, ½ cup/4oz of soya milk, 1 tbsp flaxseed/linseed oil, 9 toasted almonds and 6 ice cubes (optional). Combine all the ingredients in a blender and mix until smooth and creamy. Pour into a large glass, sprinkle with sesame seeds and serve this nutritional powerhouse cold.

Drinks

- Coffee with skimmed milk and no added sugar or syrup
- Tea with skimmed milk and no added sugar
- Herbal tea
- Filtered water
- Sugar-free smoothies
- Soya milk
- Vegetable juices
- Unsweetened fruit juices
- Diet drinks with no caffeine or added sugar
- The odd glass of red or white wine

Shopping and Cooking Guidelines

Now it's time to restock your fridge and shelves with healthy, nutritious ingredients fit for the happier, healthier and slimmer you. If you've followed the advice in this book so far, your shopping habits may already be changing. You'll be reading food labels and buying fresh rather than processed foods.

A diet high in nutrients and low in sugar, unhealthy fat, additives and preservatives is the key to good health. Although you might be buying new and different kinds of food, your new way of shopping will be just as easy as before.

Before you go shopping, make sure you aren't hungry. Hunger makes you more likely to fill your trolley with convenience and sugary foods. You might also find it helpful to sit down and list the fresh, natural ingredients you want to buy. As you review this list, you'll find that most of the foods you buy from now on are available on the outside perimeter of the store, in the fruit and vegetable or frozen food sections. With the exception of spices, olive oil, vinegar and the odd item here and there, you won't need to walk down the aisles packed with ready meals and sugar-rich foods any more.

Cupboard

- Selection of beans and pulses such as sugar-free beans, black beans, butter beans, chickpeas, haricot beans, kidney beans, mung beans, lentils, soya beans, split beans and products made from beans and pulses such as hummus.

Buying Beans

Avoid beans cooked with, or canned beans with, salt or preservatives. Choose instead ready-to-use beans cooked without animal fat or salt. Why? Beans are a fantastic source of nutrients that can help reduce cholesterol and balance your blood sugar but their nutritional value can be depleted if they are canned or cooked in fat and salt.

- Wholemeal or stone-ground bread
- Wholegrain pasta and rice
- Couscous
- Basmati rice
- Dried apricots
- Extra virgin olive oil
- Ground almonds – to replace flour in baking
- Herbs and spices of your choice – to replace salt and sugar
- Nut oils, such as walnut and macadamia
- Cold-pressed oils such as flaxseed/linseed, soya, sunflower and rapeseed
- Pesto
- Reduced-sugar baked beans
- Seeds – flaxseeds/linseeds, pumpkin seeds, sunflower seeds, hemp seeds, sesame seeds
- Sun-dried tomatoes in olive oil
- Tinned tuna and sardines
- Traditional oats
- Unsalted nuts: almonds, hazelnuts, walnuts, pecans, pine nuts, peanuts

- Bran cereal fortified with vitamin B12
- Muesli
- Vinegar – balsamic, red and white wine or flavoured vinegar
- Sweet potatoes, new potatoes or yams

Beverages

Avoid alcoholic drinks, tea, coffee, cocoa, pasteurised and/or sweetened fruit juices and fizzy drinks. Choose instead herbal teas, fresh (preferably organic) fruit and vegetable juices, mineral or filtered water. If possible, choose glass bottles.

Fridge

- Fat-free cottage cheese
- Unsweetened yoghurt, Greek yoghurt
- Skimmed milk or soya milk
- Half-fat or low-fat cheese
- Olive oil-based spreads
- Small pot of single cream or vanilla ice cream
- Organic free-range eggs – these won't contain the toxic hormones and antibiotics pumped into battery eggs
- Ready-made soups low in fat and salt
- Small bar of dark chocolate

Fruit

Choose a wide selection of fresh fruits such as apples, pears, oranges, melons, nectarines, lemons, grapes, grapefruit, pineapple, blackberries, blueberries, strawberries and so on. Avoid canned, bottled or frozen fruits with sweeteners or other additives. Fruit is always best eaten fresh because when it's processed or juiced the nutrient and fibre content decreases and the sugar and additive content increases. Don't forget to add lemons and limes to your list. Not only do they add a tangy flavour to dishes, but they can also have a balancing effect on your blood sugar levels.

Wholesomeness, quality, nutritional value and informative labelling are some of the points to consider when buying fresh fruit and vegetables. Buy fruit and vegetables that are in season – they tend to be cheaper – and buy in small amounts; twice a week or more often if possible.

Vegetables

Choose fresh and frozen vegetables rather than the canned variety. Fresh vegetables keep for about a week in the fridge; frozen keep much longer. Frozen vegetables are a good backup in case you run out of fresh during the week, and are a good choice because they're frozen at optimum ripeness. Fresh produce is sometimes harvested weeks before it arrives on the supermarket shelves and may have lost important nutrients in transit.

If you do choose canned vegetables, remove some of the salt by draining the liquid and rinsing the vegetables in water. Some vegetables are canned without the added salt. Season your vegetables with herbs, spices, lemon or vinegar to avoid adding calories from fat, such as butter.

Finally, don't get into a vegetable rut and stick with tried-and-tested favourites like peas, carrots and broccoli. There's a whole world of variety out there waiting for you. If you've never tried some of the veggies in the list below, now's your chance.

Good Vegetable Choices

- Alfalfa sprouts
- Artichoke
- Artichoke hearts
- Asparagus
- Aubergine

Good Vegetable Choices (Cont.)

- Bamboo shoots
- Beans: green, Italian, wax or yellow
- Bean sprouts
- Broccoli
- Brussels sprouts
- Cabbage
- Carrots
- Cauliflower
- Celery
- Chicory
- Chinese cabbage
- Courgettes
- Cucumber
- Greens: beet, collard, dandelion, kale, mustard or turnip
- Jicama (Mexican potato)
- Kohlrabi
- Leeks
- Lettuce: endive, escarole, leafy varieties, romaine or iceberg
- Mushrooms
- Okra
- Onions
- Parsley
- Peppers (all varieties)
- Radishes
- Sauerkraut
- Spinach
- Spring onions
- Sugar snap peas or pea pods
- Summer squash
- Swede
- Swiss chard
- Tomatoes
- Tomato juice
- Tomato purée
- Tomato sauce
- Turnips
- Vegetable juice cocktail
- Water chestnuts
- Watercress

Meat and fish

Choose lean meats that are as natural as possible, without any additives. Try to balance the amount of red and white meat you purchase, and buy lots of fish. When buying fish, avoid all fried fish, shellfish, salted fish, anchovies and fish that is canned in salt and oil. Choose instead all freshwater white fish, salmon, boiled or baked fish and water-packed tuna.

Freezer

Although it's always best to eat foods that are fresh and preferably organic, frozen vegetables and fruit are great stand-bys, as long as they're free of added salt, sugar and other additives. These foods are frozen immediately after harvesting when their nutritional content is at its highest.

Frozen fish, chicken and meats in their natural states are also fine. Natural is always best on the Menopause Diet so avoid processed products in batter or breadcrumbs as much as you can.

Now and again, when life is really hectic, you might need to eat something that takes only a few minutes to cook. The odd pre-packed frozen meal won't hurt as long as you glance at the label to ensure the list of ingredients isn't too long. Some ready meals will be quite high in fat but the light options will be high in sugar and additives so be careful.

Don't Eat Alone

Don't get into the habit of preparing one meal for yourself and another for your partner and family. There's really no need to apologise or hide the foods you buy, eat and prepare because the Menopause Diet is a basic, healthy diet that will improve everyone's health, regardless of their age and food preferences. In the first few weeks you may encounter resistance, especially if you've got children, and it's a good idea to have plenty of nutritious snacks on hand to boost energy. Things will improve once your family discover that their diet is satisfying, delicious and not restrictive (remember the 80/20 rule, *see page 29*). If you're patient and persistent, everyone's nutrition and health will improve.

Eating Out on the Menopause Diet

If you eat out a lot you can still stick to the Menopause Diet by following the guidelines below.

Don't starve yourself beforehand

It's much easier to stay in control if you've been eating sensibly throughout the day. Before you eat, drink a glass of water – you'll feel fuller and less inclined to overeat.

Try to order first

If you order first you won't be tempted or swayed by what everyone else is having. Order soup for starters; studies show that people who order soup tend to eat less overall. When choosing a soup, bear in mind that cream-based soups are higher in fat and calories than most other varieties.

Always ask how dishes are prepared

Waiters are becoming accustomed to fielding these types of question, so don't worry about pestering them. Are your dishes baked? Are they grilled? Are they prepared with butter or oil? Ask what's in the sauce; what's in the soup; what's in the dressing. Always ask for butter, gravy, sauces and salad dressings on the side. This allows you to control how much fat you eat. When ordering pasta dishes look for tomato-based sauces rather than cream-based ones as these are much lower in fat and calories. In addition, the tomato sauce (or marinara sauce) can count as a vegetable!

Take your time

Take your time over dinner and put your knife and fork down between each bite. Dining out isn't just about the food;

savour the occasion and the conversation too. If you eat your food too fast you just overload your digestive system. Stop eating when you're full – listen to the cues your body gives you. You don't have to leave your plate empty. Ask for a doggy bag so you can take half your meal home. (If you want to eat less, you could order two appetisers or an appetiser and a salad as your meal.)

Wait around 10 or 15 minutes before ordering dessert. It takes a while for your stomach to tell your brain it's had enough. If, after waiting, you absolutely can't resist ordering 'death by chocolate', make sure you split the dessert with your friends. People usually order dessert out of habit, but often a few bites are enough to satisfy even the sweetest tooth.

Choose drinks carefully

Drink water, diet fizzy drinks or unsweetened tea or coffee instead of regular fizzy drinks or alcoholic beverages. This will save a lot of calories. If you're worried about drinking too much alcohol, stick to spritzers. Mixing some sparkling water with your white wine means you can drink twice as much without having to worry.

Sample Recipes

Mixed Grain Porridge

This low-calorie, low-fat, high-fibre porridge makes the perfect start to the day. It's also rich in phytoestrogens, antioxidants and omega 3.

Serves 3

425ml (¾ pint) soya milk
30g (1oz) millet grains
30g (1oz) barley flakes
30g (1oz) rolled oats

To serve
Fromage frais
Honey
Chopped dried fruits such as apricots and cranberries
1 tsp pumpkin seeds and almonds

1. Pour the milk into a saucepan and bring to the boil, then add the millet, barley and oats. Reduce the heat and simmer for 10 minutes, stirring occasionally until the mixture is thin and soft.
2. Spoon into a porridge bowl. Top with fromage frais and a little honey and sprinkle over the dried fruit, seeds and almonds.

Raspberry Pot

This is low in calories and fat, and high in fibre, antioxidants and protein. You'll also be getting phytoestrogens from the raspberries and omega 3 from the walnuts.

Serves 4

30–40 fresh raspberries
425ml (¾ pint) low-fat natural yoghurt

To serve
4 tbsp honey
30g (1oz) chopped, unsalted walnuts

1. Arrange the raspberries snugly at the bottom of 4 glasses or glass bowls. Spoon the yoghurt over the raspberries and chill for 10 minutes.
2. To serve, drizzle 1 tbsp honey over each dessert and sprinkle with chopped walnuts.

Bean and Escarole Salad

This salad offers plenty of fibre, protein, magnesium and hormone-balancing phytoestrogens. If you can't find soya beans, try cooked, shelled edamame or pinto beans. Kelp granules are available at health food stores.

Serves 4

Dressing
1 tbsp flax oil
1 tbsp water
1 tbsp soy sauce or tamari
1 tbsp lemon juice
2 tsp Dijon mustard
1 tsp kelp granules

Salad
425g (15oz) tin soya beans, drained, rinsed and patted dry
   on paper towels
½ medium red pepper, seeded and cut into 0.5cm (¼-inch)
   dice (about ½ cup/4 oz)
¼ cup/2 oz chopped fresh parsley leaves
2 cups/16 oz finely shredded escarole
1 small avocado, peeled, pitted and cut into 0.5cm (¼-inch) dice

1. Combine all the dressing ingredients in a small bowl
   with a whisk and set aside.
2. Gently mix the soya beans, pepper and parsley together
   in a medium bowl. Add the dressing, toss gently and
   set aside for at least 5 minutes or up to an hour.
3. When ready to serve, divide the escarole between
   4 small bowls. Gently mix the avocado into the bean
   salad. Spoon some bean salad over each portion of
   escarole. Serve immediately.

Lentil Soup

This nourishing and satisfying soup is rich in fibre and phytoestrogens.

Serves 2–3

115g (4oz) red lentils
425ml (15fl oz) vegetable stock
120ml (4fl oz) water
½ an onion
1 clove garlic
½ tsp sunflower oil
Pinch ground cumin
2 lemon wedges

1. Pour the lentils into a pan, add the stock and water and bring to boiling point. Simmer for 30 minutes, removing any scum that rises to the surface with a wooden spoon.
2. Peel and chop the onion. Peel and crush the garlic. Heat the oil in a non-stick frying pan over a moderate heat. Fry the garlic and onion until brown.
3. Add the cumin to the lentils and stir well. Serve the soup in individual bowls and garnish with the onion and garlic mixture and lemon wedges. Wholemeal bread makes a good accompaniment.

Beans with Garlic and Tomatoes

This recipe is packed with phytoestrogens, fibre, antioxidants and protein. The baby spinach garnish provides extra iron and vitamin C.

Serves 6

395g (14oz) dried butterbeans, soaked in water overnight
90ml (3fl oz) extra virgin olive oil
2 large onions, chopped
3 garlic cloves, sliced thinly
1 red pepper, deseeded and diced
1 celery stick, trimmed, rinsed and sliced
2 carrots, sliced thinly
1 tbsp dried oregano
1 tbsp dried thyme
395g (14oz) tin tomatoes, chopped
2 tbsp tomato purée, diluted with 450ml (16fl oz) hot water
½ tsp sugar
Sea salt
4 tbsp finely chopped flat-leaf parsley

To serve
Baby spinach

1. Preheat the oven to 180°C/Gas Mark 4.
2. Rinse the beans, put them in a saucepan with plenty of water, cover and boil for about 30 minutes until almost cooked. Drain.
3. Heat the oil in a saucepan, add the onions and sauté until golden. Add the garlic and fry for 2 minutes. Add the pepper, celery, carrots and dried herbs and sauté for 5–6 minutes. Add the tomatoes, diluted

purée and sugar. Cover and cook for 10 minutes. Add
the beans, season and cook gently for 15 minutes.
4. Stir in the parsley, transfer to an ovenproof dish and
cook for 30 minutes or until brown around the edges.
Serve hot or at room temperature, sprinkled with
baby spinach.

Spinach and Tofu Salad

This delicious salad is low in calories and fat and rich in iron,
antioxidants and phytoestrogens.

Serves 1

170g (6oz) tofu
4 tbsp lemon juice
1 tbsp powdered ginger
1 tbsp black pepper
115g (4oz) fresh spinach
70g (2½ oz) carrots, sliced
55g (2oz) green pepper, sliced

For the dressing
1 tbsp soy sauce
1 tbsp white vinegar
1 tbsp water
1 tbsp olive oil
1 garlic clove, crushed

1. Cut the tofu into chunks and combine in a bowl with
the lemon juice, ginger and black pepper. Place in the
oven on a lightly greased baking tray and cook until
brown (325°C/Gas Mark 3 for 20–40 minutes).

2. Combine the spinach, carrots and green pepper. Mix together the soy sauce, white vinegar, water, olive oil and garlic and pour this dressing over the salad. Add the tofu and toss well. Serve with a slice of wholemeal bread.

Salmon Dinner

This is light in fat and calories and rich in antioxidants and omega 3.

Serves 1

120ml (4fl oz) skimmed milk
115g (4oz) salmon
1 lemon wedge
85g (3oz) broccoli, divided into florets
1 clove garlic, chopped
1 tbsp flaxseed/linseed oil

1. Heat the milk in a frying pan and add the salmon. Poach the salmon on high heat for 5–7 minutes. Check the middle of the fish to see that it's done. Sprinkle with fresh lemon juice.
2. Put the broccoli in a steamer with the garlic and steam for 10 minutes. Sprinkle with flaxseed/linseed oil. Serve the salmon and broccoli with new potatoes or a baked potato.

Fish Parcels

These delicious parcels are low in fat and calories and a good source of protein, omega 3, antioxidants and sulphurous compounds to boost your liver.

Serves 2

2 fillets of oily fish like salmon or trout, skinned
2 small heads of bok choy
1 celery stick, trimmed
2 large onions
2 large brown mushrooms
2 tbsp oyster sauce

1. Wash and dry the fish and cut into 2cm (¾-inch) crosswise strips. Cut the bok choy in half lengthwise. Divide it between 2 pieces of greaseproof paper and place the fish on top.
2. Cut the celery into diagonal 2cm (¾-inch) pieces and the onions in half, then into thick lengthwise strips. Slice the mushrooms thinly. Divide the vegetables between each fish parcel. Spoon 1 tbsp of oyster sauce over each. Wrap up to make a parcel and then place on a rack over a pan of boiling water. If you have a bamboo steamer, you can use it over a wok or pan. Cover and steam for 5 minutes or until the fish is cooked.
3. To serve, cut a cross in the paper to reveal the contents. Serve with brown rice for extra energy, fibre and a good dose of calming B vitamins.

Vegetable Stew

An antioxidant-rich and energy-boosting stew.

Serves 2–3

1 large onion, peeled and chopped
1 large clove garlic, peeled and chopped
1 tbsp olive oil
170g (6oz) fresh spinach, chopped
395g (14oz) tin chickpeas
395g (14oz) tin tomatoes, chopped
4 or 5 fresh tomatoes, chopped
70g (2½ oz) raisins
2 new potatoes, peeled and chopped
85g (3oz) brown rice
Sea salt to taste

1. Fry the onion and garlic in the olive oil. Add the
   spinach and cook until limp, then add the rest of the
   ingredients, except the sea salt.
2. Cook for 45 minutes or until the potatoes are soft and
   can be pricked by a fork. You may need to add a little
   water if the stew gets too thick.
3. Add the sea salt and serve.

Spinach-stuffed Chicken Breasts

These are low in calories and fat and a good source of antioxidants and iron.

Serves 4

125g (4½ oz) fresh spinach
55g (2oz) low-fat cream cheese or fromage frais
Sea salt and pepper
1 onion, grated
1 tbsp grated lemon rind
55g (2oz) chestnut mushrooms, chopped finely
4 skinless chicken breasts (about 140g/5oz each)
1 large potato, parboiled

1. Preheat the oven to 190°C/Gas Mark 5.
2. Put the spinach and cream cheese or fromage frais into a food processor and whiz until smooth. Season with sea salt and a pinch of pepper and transfer to a bowl.
3. Heat a frying pan and dry-fry the onion for 5 minutes until soft and brown. Add the lemon rind and mushrooms and fry for a further 5 minutes to extract the juice from the mushrooms. Stir into the spinach mixture.
4. Make a cut along the length of each chicken breast and open up to form a pocket. Spoon a little of the spinach mixture into each pocket.
5. Slice the potato and arrange in a layer in an ovenproof dish, overlapping slightly. Place the chicken breasts on top of the potatoes and season. Cover the chicken with foil to prevent it from over-browning. Bake for 45 minutes. Serve with roasted red onion and tomatoes.

Baked Stuffed Apples

Serves 2

2 good-sized cooking apples
Stuffing suggestions: dates, cinnamons, raisins
1 tbsp honey or sugar-free jam

1. Core the apples and slit the skins in a ring around the middle. Stuff the core with your chosen filling and honey or jam.
2. Bake at 200°C/Gas Mark 6 for 50 minutes or until the fruit is tender and serve hot or cold.

Fruit Kebabs

If you don't find fruit all that appealing, here's a way to make it more interesting. Buy a pack of wooden skewers from your supermarket. Cut fruit into 2.5cm (1-inch) squares and thread on the skewers. Try alternating chunks of pineapple with melon, peach, apricots, bananas and grapes. Eat with a handful of roasted almonds for a nutritious and satisfying snack.

Bluestraw Fruit Smoothie

This is an excellent source of antioxidants and essential fats. It's high in fibre too, so great for detox.

Serves 1

8 fresh or frozen strawberries
1 banana
70g (2½ oz) fresh or frozen blueberries
1 tbsp flaxseed/linseed oil
6 whole blanched almonds
2 tbsp oat bran
120ml (4fl oz) skimmed milk or orange juice

1. Halve the strawberries and peel the banana, cutting it in half if it's big. Blend the strawberries, banana, blueberries, flaxseed/linseed oil, almonds and oat bran until smooth. Add the milk or orange juice and blend again. Serve chilled.

You could vary this by using phytoestrogen-rich soya milk and playing around with different combinations of fruit to a get a good mix of nutrients. Try mangoes, pineapples and raspberries or banana, peach and berries – delicious.

How to Lose Weight Naturally at Midlife

The Menopause Diet and detox guidelines will help stabilise your blood sugar levels and hormones, so you may find you start to lose weight without even trying. If, however, the pounds aren't shifting as quickly as you'd like, this chapter will give you lots of tips to help them melt away.

As you work through this chapter, never forget the first and most important rule of the Menopause Diet: healthy eating and *not* dieting to lose weight is the key. If you want to lose weight, you need to eat. Your body needs a regular supply of nutrients from all food groups so it can beat food cravings, boost your metabolism and burn fat.

If you're eating healthily and exercising and still not losing excess weight, you should visit your doctor to rule out any underlying medical condition, such as diabetes, an underactive thyroid or polycystic ovaries. Weight loss is tougher with these conditions but not impossible, and you'll need to work closely with your doctor to find the best diet and treatment programme.

Do I Really Need to Lose Weight?

Being overweight can increase your risk of heart disease and cancer but your risk is only partly determined by the number you see on your bathroom scales. To get a fuller picture of how your weight will affect your health, you need to know your body mass index (BMI), and your waist-hip ratio.

Find your BMI

Right now, the best tool for deciding if your current weight is healthy is the BMI. Essentially, the BMI is a formula that relates to body fat. It's better at predicting the risk of disease than body weight alone. To find your BMI, measure your height in metres and multiply the figure by itself, giving your height squared. Then measure your weight in kilograms. Divide the weight by the height squared. For a woman measuring 1.6m (5 feet 3 inches) and weighing 65kg (10 stone), the calculation would be: 1.6 x 1.6 = 2.56. Then 65 divided by 2.56 = 25.39. A BMI of between 18.3 and 24.9 means you are an ideal weight, according to the World Health Organization. If your BMI is over 25, this is considered too heavy and if your BMI is under 18, this is considered underweight.

The BMI can also be used to help determine your weight loss goal. If your BMI is over 25, calculate the weight you would need to be to have a BMI of 25. Then subtract your answer from your current weight to find your weight loss goal. Is this weight loss realistic? Much depends on your age and your circumstances. You may have to settle for a 5 or 10 per cent weight loss from your current weight – even this change would be enough to prevent diabetes and heart disease. If your goal is a high number – say over 23kg (50lb) – consider it as a long-term goal, something to be accomplished over the next three years. Break it down into manageable stages, such as aiming to lose 9kg (20lb) a year. Whatever your goal, weight loss of one or two pounds a week

is a realistic and healthy expectation and sets you on the path
to finding your natural weight.

Calculate your waist-hip ratio

Grab a tape measure and measure your waist at its narrowest
point, when your stomach is relaxed. Next, measure the
circumference of your hips at their widest, in other words
where your bottom sticks out the most. Finally, divide your
waist measurement by your hip measurement. A healthy target
is 0.8 or less. At this ratio you're not carrying excess weight
around your middle.

Do take your body shape into account when setting your
weight loss goals. Apple and pear shapes are definitely not
equal when it comes to the risk of developing diabetes and
other diseases. If you're an apple, the risk is higher (*see
Chapter 2, page 19*).

Natural Treatments for Weight Loss

If the numbers say you need to lose weight, here are some
natural strategies that will help you successfully lose weight – and
keep it off. You won't find a quick fix here. The only way to lose
weight permanently is to change your eating habits according to
the Menopause Diet guidelines in Chapter 3, and make these
guidelines an eating plan for life. Sustainable weight loss has to
be gradual and it will take time. You should aim to lose no more
than two pounds per week. This can seem slow and frustrating,
but research has shown that the gradual approach to weight
loss works; and the weight will stay off for good.

Foods and supplements

If you're trying to lose weight you should increase your intake
of certain nutrient-rich foods. If you're following the

Fat-fighting Foods

Almonds: Studies presented at the 2005 Experimental Biology Conference in California showed that adding almonds to your diet may contribute to greater satiety and prevent weight gain. The researchers hypothesised that the high levels of fibre and protein could be responsible.

Apples: Apples contain pectin, a chemical also found in most berries and fresh fruit. The pectin is in the cell walls of most fruits, especially apples, and limits the amount of fat your cells can absorb.

Avocado: Studies have shown that essential fatty acids and proteins such as those found in avocado boost metabolism and promote weight loss.

Bananas: These are a good food source of magnesium, a mineral critical for energy production and proper nerve function. Magnesium also promotes muscle relaxation and helps the body produce and use insulin. It's also the key to calcium absorption; a correct balance between the two minerals is important for weight loss.

Barley: This is a good source of soluble fibre which research has shown is important for weight loss.

Blueberries: These are a fantastic source of vitamin C. Studies have shown that sufficient vitamin C intake is crucial for weight management.

Broccoli: Study after study links calcium and weight loss. Broccoli is not only high in calcium but also loaded with vitamin C, which boosts calcium absorption, and isoflavones (see Chapter 7, page 147).

Cinnamon: An increasing number of studies show that cinnamon contains substances that can help the body convert sugar into energy so it's less likely to be stored as fat.

Garlic: This contains a substance called allicin. Research has shown that allicin has a significant protective quality to cells that help to reduce fatty deposits.

Grapefruit: It's thought that the unique chemical properties of fat-fighting, vitamin C-packed citrus fruit help reduce insulin levels, preventing fat storage and promoting weight loss.

Hot peppers: Eating hot peppers can speed up your metabolism and cool your cravings, researchers have found. Here's why: capsaicin (a chemical found in jalapeño and cayenne peppers) temporarily stimulates your body to release more stress hormones. This speeds up your metabolism and causes you to burn more calories.

Lean turkey: Turkey is a good source of CLA (conjugated linoleic acid). Recent research published in the Journal of Nutrition confirms that CLA helps long-term body fat reduction and so promotes weight loss.

Oatmeal: This is a good source of cholesterol-fighting, fat-soluble fibre that boosts metabolism and keeps you feeling fuller for longer.

Fat-fighting Foods (Cont.)

Odd glass of red wine: Although rich in calories, the odd glass of wine now and again can benefit weight loss. It seems that grape seeds contain substances that have an inhibiting effect on weight gain.

Oily fish: Salmon, mackerel, herring and other oily fish are a great source of essential fats that have been shown to be essential for weight loss.

Pears: Overweight women who ate the equivalent of three small pears a day lost more weight on a low-calorie diet than women who didn't add fruit to their diet, according to researchers from the State University of Rio de Janeiro. Fruit-eaters also ate fewer calories overall. So, next time you need to satisfy a sugar craving, reach for this low-calorie, high-fibre snack. You'll feel full for longer and eat less.

Quinoa: This is a great source of complete protein. Countless studies have shown that protein can help boost metabolism, burn fat and build lean muscle tissue.

Seaweed (kelp): Research suggests that kelp contains a rich supply of nutrients that can help restore hormonal balance and boost metabolism.

Soya beans: These contain lecithin, a chemical that shields your cells from accumulating fat. This chemical also breaks down fatty deposits in your body.

Spinach: Research continues to confirm that diets high in nutrient-rich vegetables are associated with a reduced risk of weight gain. Spinach provides the nutritional support needed for healthy, effective weight loss.

Sunflower seeds: These seeds are a powerhouse of nutritious protein, vitamins, minerals and nutrients that boost energy and metabolism and promote weight loss.

Walnuts: Research has shown that 30g (1oz) of walnuts a day improves the lipid profile of patients with type two diabetes and reduces the risk of obesity.

Menopause Diet you should be getting enough of these already, but listed above are some good examples of low-calorie, nutrient-rich foods that can help you lose weight.

When it comes to weight loss, a multivitamin and mineral is highly recommended to offer you a little extra nutritional insurance. A good one will provide you with the recommended daily amounts of all the key vitamins and minerals you need to keep your metabolism (fat burning) humming along. (*See Chapter 7 for more advice on multivitamins.*)

Although all nutrients are important for weight loss, some are particularly useful. Being deficient in any of them could hinder your weight loss plans so you need to make sure your diet and supplement programme is rich in them. Here are the key players:

Vitamin B

B vitamins are important for weight loss because they're involved in energy production and fat metabolism, and help you digest your food better. If digestion is good you're more likely to use your food efficiently rather than storing it as fat. It's best to get your B vitamins from your diet. Foods such as whole grains, nuts, fish, vegetables and low-fat dairy products are rich in B vitamins. However, if you think you may be deficient the best way to make sure you're getting enough vitamin B is a good B complex supplement.

Calcium

This important bone-building mineral is often missing from diets designed for weight loss, but research has shown that it is in fact important for losing weight. It seems that calcium stored in fat cells plays a crucial role in regulating how fat is stored and broken down by the body. It's thought that the more calcium there is in a fat cell, the more fat it will burn. So if you want to lose weight, don't immediately jettison dairy from your diet; the key is low-fat rather than high-fat dairy. Other good sources of calcium include leafy green vegetables. You should be aiming for 1,000–1,200mg of calcium each day. If you want to use calcium supplements, it's important to choose those with added vitamin D, zinc and magnesium, as these help the body to absorb calcium. Calcium citrate is more easily absorbed than calcium carbonate.

Chromium

This mineral is needed for the metabolism of sugar. Without it, insulin is less effective in controlling blood sugar levels, making it harder to burn off food as fuel so that more is stored as fat. Chromium may also help control levels of fat and cholesterol in the blood, according to one study. Good food sources of chromium include whole grains, bananas, carrots, cabbage, mushrooms and strawberries. If you want to take a chromium supplement, most people take 50–200mcg a day of organic chelated chromium picolinate rather than standard chromium supplements that are less easy to absorb.

Manganese

This mineral helps with the absorption of fats and works to stabilise blood sugar levels. It also functions in many enzymes, including those involved in burning energy. Make sure your multivitamin and mineral contains manganese. Foods rich in manganese include green leafy vegetables, pecans, pulses and whole grains.

Magnesium

It's important that this mineral is in good supply as it aids the production of insulin and helps regulate blood sugar levels. Foods rich in magnesium include green leafy vegetables, nuts and seeds and soya beans. If you want to supplement with magnesium, the recommended daily intake is in the region of 300mg.

Co-enzyme Q10

This is needed for energy production, and studies have also shown that it can help with weight loss. Good food sources include sardines, soya oil, whole grains and mackerel. If you want to take a supplement, ideally you should do so under the guidance of a nutritional therapist. The usual dose is two 60mg capsules twice a day.

Zinc

This mineral is important because it can help control appetite; a deficiency can cause a loss of taste and smell. Make sure your multivitamin and mineral contains zinc, and include more zinc-rich foods in your diet, such as green leafy vegetables, nuts, seeds, whole grains and eggs. If you don't think you're getting enough zinc you may want to take a daily 15g supplement, but no more than this as high levels can make you vulnerable to infection.

Other nutritional supplements

Here are some other nutritional supplements that are often recommended to help weight loss:

- Potassium: important in the production of energy
- EFAs (essential fatty acids): for appetite control
- Psyllium husks: for fibre to promote a fuller feeling
- Kelp: contains minerals that can help with weight loss
- Lecithin capsules: can help break down fat
- Spirulina: can help stabilise blood sugar
- Vitamin C: to speed up a slow metabolism
- Boron: to speed up the burning of calories (raisins and onions are good sources)
- The amino acids L-Ornithine, L-Arginine and L-Lysine:

research has shown that weight loss can be improved with a combination of these

If you want to take any nutritional, herbal or fat-fighting supplement to help you lose weight, such as Siberian ginseng, garcinia cambogia, fennel or fenugreek, you need to consult your doctor and a trained dietitian or nutritionist first. Certain herbal supplements can be toxic in large doses. Ephedra is a popular ingredient in many over the counter weight loss formulations but it has been shown to cause irregular heartbeats, strokes, hypertension and anxiety – hardly a harmless profile, so best avoided.

Unless your doctor feels that your weight carries a serious risk to your health or that you could benefit from a short-term dieting drug, like Reductil, steer clear of slimming drugs of any kind. What you need is permanent weight loss, and the drawback of slimming drugs is that they are like diets: they don't work in the long term. The best way to lose weight is to gain control of your eating habits and increase the amount of exercise you get.

Find an Exercise you Enjoy

If you don't lead an active lifestyle, now is the time to get moving. The benefits of exercise for women approaching menopause cannot be exaggerated. Regular exercise can help balance your hormones and reduce your risk of heart disease, diabetes, cancer, osteoporosis and high blood pressure. It helps to keep your bowels working efficiently so toxins are cleared quickly, and also boosts your immunity, energy levels, libido and self-esteem. And we haven't even come to the weight loss bit yet.

Exercise speeds up your metabolism and burns calories. By building up muscle it helps your body burn calories even when at rest. With all these benefits exercise simply has to be an essential part of your Menopause Diet programme.

Be careful not to launch yourself into a vigorous exercise routine. Instead, begin slowly with mild exercise and then gradually build up, especially if you've not been active for a while. Walk instead of run; swim or cycle at an easy pace and so on. Then, once you feel stronger, you can increase the intensity and length of your workout but, as before, make sure you do this gradually.

> **WARNING**
>
> If you are overweight, have high blood pressure or a pre-existing medical condition make sure you check with your doctor before beginning an exercise routine.

Your exercise prescription

Once you know it's safe to exercise, exercise safely! Use your common sense and listen to your body. You will probably experience some discomfort or even soreness after a session when you first get going, but there shouldn't be any pain, fainting, dizziness, shortness of breath or nausea. So don't overdo it. If something doesn't feel right, STOP immediately and talk to your doctor.

Be sure to wear loose, comfortable clothing when exercising, and make sure your shoes offer the correct support. Drink plenty of water before, during and after your workout, even if you aren't thirsty, and have light snacks to hand in case you get a sudden dip in energy. Finally, pay attention to your breathing when you're exercising. Try to prevent it becoming quick and shallow. You should breathe in deeply through your nose and out through your mouth.

To improve your health and quality of life you don't need to join a gym or run the marathon; you need just 30 minutes of activity per day. And you don't have to get all 30 minutes at once – your exercise can be spread throughout the day and include activities such as climbing stairs, a brisk walk or cleaning the house. Any activity counts. You just need to get 30 minutes a day most days of the week. If you don't think you're getting your 30 minutes, find ways to get there: park further away from work so you've got to walk; take the stairs instead of the lift; carry your shopping home; wash your car by hand; mow the lawn. In the long run these simple changes can help you prevent health complications and feel better about yourself.

Whatever you decide to do, make sure you enjoy it. Studies show that exercise dropouts often punish themselves with routines they don't enjoy. So if you hate jogging or swimming, don't do it. Find an exercise you enjoy so that you can stick with it. It doesn't have to be a traditional exercise or class – if dancing, rambling, horse riding or boxing are things you enjoy, make them part of your exercise routine. If you do skip a workout, don't let it derail your exercise prescription. If you're working out five times a week for 30 minutes, giving yourself a day or two off now and again isn't going to undo the good you've done.

Half an hour a day is a small price to pay for your health and wellbeing. There really is no excuse now. Taking time out of your day for exercise can take inches from your waistline and add years – healthy, energetic years – to your future.

Before and after exercising

You should start an exercise session with a gradual warm-up period. During this time (about 5–10 minutes), you should slowly stretch your muscles first, and then gradually increase your level of activity. For example, begin walking slowly and then pick up the pace. You might also want to have a light snack 20 or so minutes before exercising as this will encourage your body to burn fat, not muscle, when you start moving.

After you've finished exercising, cool down for about 5–10 minutes. Again, stretch your muscles and let your heart rate slow down gradually. You can use the same stretches as in the warm-up period.

Sample exercise plan

Walking

Walking is great. No expertise or equipment is required, you can do it any time and it's free! What's more, provided you do it regularly and for long enough, walking can be just as beneficial as any of the more vigorous activities, such as jogging.

To start, take a 10-minute walk twice a day. To extend yourself gradually:

- Walk every day
- Walk for longer
- Walk faster
- Walk and swing your arms at the same time
- Walk up one or two gentle slopes
- Walk up steeper slopes

Ideally, aim to walk briskly (swinging your arms) for 30 minutes each day. This should include at least one reasonably steep slope. Please note that this may take you several months to achieve, so don't be in a hurry. Remember, exercise is for life!

Swimming

For most people, especially those who are very overweight, swimming is even better than walking. Start by going to the pool twice a week for a gentle 15-minute swim, then gradually increase the length of your swim and your work rate while in the water. Aim to build up to about 30 minutes a day, or 45 minutes twice a week.

Cycling/cycle-machine, trampoline or jogging

Start with a short, easy routine – 10–15 minutes per day – and work up to about 30 minutes a day. Increase your work rate gradually, without ever straining yourself. If jogging, invest in a good pair of running shoes that offer cushioned support. You'll also need a good sports bra for all these activities. When exercising, keep your breathing steady and never get so out of breath that you can't hold a conversation.

Toning exercises

Once you've got going with your 30 minutes of activity, you should also think about including some strength-bearing activities two or three times a week for 10–15 minutes. This is because the more muscle you have the more calories you burn and the better your blood sugar balance, even when you're not exercising. This is especially important once you hit 40 as the average woman loses about half a pound of muscle a year and gains one and a half pounds of body fat. Unfortunately, the fat tends to appear in the most annoying of places: the back roll, the flapping arms and larger waist line. But clever strength exercises – lifting weights, yoga, Pilates, t'ai chi – can reap great streamlining rewards. If you aren't into any of these, carry your shopping bags, lift your kids or do some sit-ups and press-ups as you watch television. Find ways in your daily life to use your muscles more.

You could also make time every other day to do the following toning exercises. While you won't eliminate the bulges entirely, you'll firm up muscle tone and prevent further fat gain. Plus you'll feel the benefits in less than a month. Just remember to warm up with a few gentle stretches beforehand (*see page 113*).

Toning the chest

Unfortunately, pregnancy and/or the laws of gravity mean that your breasts start to droop as you get older. Wearing a properly fitted bra is essential to make the most of your figure, but you could also give your breasts a helping hand by strengthening your pectorals – the muscles that support them. Try this exercise:

Lie on your back with your feet flat on the floor and arms bent at 90 'egrees. Hold a tin of beans or soup or a light dumbbell in each hand and push the weights up so they are directly over your chest. Then slowly lower the weights, with your elbows out to the side, lightly touching the floor. Don't lock your elbows. Do four sets of 10 repetitions.

Toning the bottom

This area also has a tendency to droop over the years. Squats will make your bottom more pert and your thighs firmer. To squat, stand with your feet shoulder width apart, bend your knees and slowly start to sit down. Once your bottom is nearly in line with your knees, slowly push up into a standing position, squeezing your bottom as you do so. Do two sets of 10 repetitions.

Toning the upper arms

Sit on the edge of a chair and place your hands on the seat with fingers over the edge and elbows pointing behind you.

Lift your bottom off the seat and walk one step forwards. With feet hip distance apart, lower your bottom by bending your elbows to 90 degrees. Aim for 20 repetitions.

Toning the tummy

During menopause, you are more likely to gain fat around the midriff, together with a loss of muscle tone. The following tips will help trim and tone this area.

The best way to burn fat around the stomach is with regular aerobic exercise, such as brisk walking, swimming, cycling, dancing or jogging. Aerobic workouts are very important because they can, if done properly, increase your metabolism for 24 hours or more. This means that you're less likely to store any excess calories as fat on your tummy. Plus, you're more likely to burn off excess body fat in the process.

You need to combine regular aerobic exercises with toning exercises, such as the abdominal lift and basic crunch. For the abdominal lift:

- Stand up straight with legs spaced 30cm (1 foot) apart and place your hands on your thighs.
- Inhale deeply then exhale fully. Keeping the air out of your lungs, pull your abdominal muscles in. Hold for a count of 10.
- Release, inhale and relax.
- Repeat on an empty stomach three times a day.

For the basic crunch:

- Lie flat on your back with your knees bent and feet flat on the floor. Place your hands lightly behind your head for support.
- Using your abdominal muscles lift your shoulders a few

inches off the ground, pause briefly and return to start position.
- Complete at least one set of 10–12 repetitions. Rest for a minute between sets.

Although the crunch is the single best exercise for toning the abdominal wall, it doesn't always flatten the stomach as much as we'd like. To do that, you must perform the plank as well:

- Lie flat on your stomach and place your hands on either side of your chest, as if ready to perform a press-up, although your elbows should be tucked into your sides.
- Keeping your back perfectly flat, push yourself up onto your knees so that your upper body is off the floor, with your hands and knees acting as support.
- Keeping your back flat, pull in your belly button as much as possible, as if to suck it in close to the spine. Aim to maintain a normal breathing pattern and hold this position for 10–60 seconds.
- Rest, lie flat then repeat twice.

Tips for a Flat Tum

Watch your posture: Poor posture and slumping as you walk can make even a flat stomach look saggy. Good posture has nothing to do with the old-school rigidity of pulling in your stomach and puffing your chest out. It's about keeping your body upright and your stomach firm by using the muscles that run along your spine and legs.

Eat strawberries: They are a wonderful low-calorie, nutrient-dense snack packed with fibre, vitamins, minerals and antioxidants – all nutrients essential for weight loss. They also have a very low glycaemic index (GI) rating. This means they produce only a small rise in blood glucose, keeping insulin levels steady and reducing hunger and bloating between meals – all key factors in controlling your weight and keeping that tummy flat.

Deal with bloating: If bloating is making your stomach look flabby and you feel heavy, see the tips in Chapter 8, page 156.

Tips for a Flat Tum (Cont.)

Avoid alcohol: Any alcoholic drink can add to the size of your stomach because it causes bloating and is dense in calories. Every gram of alcohol contains the same number of calories as a gram of butter, and almost twice as many as a gram of most other carbohydrates or proteins. Like other calorie-packed foods it promotes weight gain. If you can't give it up completely, bear in mind that beer drinkers tend to have the highest waist-hip ratios and wine drinkers have the slimmest waistlines.

Find a fitness trainer: If you feel you need an extra boost you could enlist the help of a professional trainer and say that you want to focus on toning the stomach area. You don't need to go for a regular weekly slot; one or two sessions should be enough to teach you some basics. A qualified fitness trainer can help you achieve your health and fitness goals, and in less time than you might imagine. If gyms and personal trainers aren't your scene, buy a book or video with plenty of advice about toning the stomach area.

Dress carefully: If you've got a flabby tummy and want to disguise it, make sure clothes skim your body but don't cling to it, and that tops hang from above or on your tummy rather than underneath it.

How to keep exercising

Only a third of those who begin an exercise programme are still exercising by the end of their first year. The good news is that with some planning and strategies, you can beat the dropout odds and make a successful transition to a lifestyle that incorporates exercise.

Find a fitness partner: Studies show that exercise adherence is generally greater if the family or a friend is included in the commitment to exercise. Find a walking partner, play tennis with your spouse or go rollerblading with the kids.

Start an exercise log or journal: This is an excellent way to chart your progress and provide motivation. Nothing beats the feeling of success as you read through your accomplishments. Exercise logs can take many forms: a calendar to record your workouts; a daily journal to record your feelings and goals; a computerised exercise log or one purchased at a book shop. The key is to select a log or journal that fits your needs and provides you with the kind of information that is meaningful to you.

Schedule your workouts: Exercise must be a priority in order to establish it as a lifestyle practice. Make time for your workouts and schedule them on your daily calendar or planner.

Toss your scales: Ask yourself, 'How often has stepping on the scales in the morning ruined my day?' If your answer is 'often', consider whether or not you should give that little machine such power over you. The fact is that exercise shouldn't revolve around a number on a scale. It should be about making a commitment to your health and wellbeing. Weight loss is a natural side-effect of that commitment.

Dress the part: Wear comfortable clothes appropriate for exercising. They will help you feel like working out. If you go to a gym, put your exercise gear in a bag and set it beside the front door the night before. When it's time to head out, all you have to do is grab your bag.

Entertain yourself: If you exercise alone, consider using a portable music device to listen to your favourite music or audio books during your workout. Many pieces of exercise equipment have racks that hold reading material. If you exercise at home, turn on some music or bring the television within viewing range.

More Tips for Keeping Motivated

- Change your activities and exercise routine so you don't get bored. Doing housework may not be fun but it does get you moving! So does gardening and walking the dog.
- If you can't set aside one block of time, do short activities during the day, such as three 10-minute walks.
- Create opportunities for activity, such as parking your car further away, taking the stairs instead of the lift, or walking down the hall to talk to a colleague instead of using e-mail.

More Tips for Keeping Motivated (Cont.)

- Don't let the cold weather keep you on the sofa! You can still find activities to do in the winter like exercising to a workout video or joining a sports club. Or get a head start on your spring cleaning by choosing active indoor chores like window washing or reorganising wardrobes.
- If you have children, make time to play with them outside. Set a positive and active example!
- Read fitness books or magazines to inspire you.
- Make exercise non-negotiable. Think of exercise as something you do without question, like brushing your teeth or going to work.

Stress-proof your diet

Do you turn to sugary, fatty food when you feel stressed, low, tired, sad, angry, guilty or lonely? If so, you need to find ways to stress-proof your diet to help you at times when you know you are vulnerable to comfort eating.

One of the best ways to stress-proof your diet is to plan ahead. Every day, plan an eating schedule for the following day. Make sure every meal has a good balance of carbohydrate, protein and fat to keep you feeling fuller for longer and less likely to crave sugary snacks. You should also plan snacks to keep your blood sugar levels up so you aren't tempted to search for pick-me-ups. Plan a mid-morning snack around three hours after breakfast, ideally a protein source like yoghurt and a piece of fruit. Eat your mid-afternoon snack about three hours after lunch. This should include protein as well as carbohydrate and be low in fat. Examples include soup with crackers, cottage cheese and fruit, low-fat yoghurt and fruit. Have a light dinner and a snack before bedtime to prevent the night-time munchies. Without planning, you make yourself vulnerable to overeating, especially from about 3pm to midnight.

Planning ahead need not become another stress. Make out healthy shopping lists; keep healthy snacks in your desk at work and in the cupboard at home; and find out which local restaurants serve healthy foods so you can opt to meet friends there.

Sometimes, however much you plan ahead, things change. You have to be able to adapt your eating routine to our fast-paced society. Keep your kitchen well stocked with emergency healthy foods like soup, beans, canned veggies and low-fat frozen meals. Fresh fruits and vegetables are good to nibble on whenever you feel hungry. If you find your routine totally disrupted due to, say, a flight cancellation or a visit to a friend in hospital, help yourself to fruit, yoghurt and made-to-order sandwiches rather than high-fat alternatives.

If your cupboard and fridge are stocked with sugary snacks, throw them out and replace them with fruits, nuts, seeds and healthier snacks. Sugary carbohydrates – such as cakes, chocolate, crisps, sweets and pastries – are the foods we often crave because they send blood sugar levels rocketing, giving us an instant energy boost. However, this boost is short lived as it leads to an overproduction of insulin followed by a dip in blood sugar, leaving us tired and craving the foods all over again.

It might also help to keep a food diary. Writing down exactly what you eat and drink isn't about calorie counting but about awareness. A food diary can help you identify situations and foods that trigger comfort eating. Once you become aware of them you can start to deal with them. For example, if you like to eat while watching television, try knitting, drinking a glass of water, riding an exercise bike or writing some thank you notes instead. If your cravings are triggered by being in the kitchen, go for a walk or do some gardening. If you're out shopping try to avoid cafés and restaurants. At parties steer clear of the buffet table and use your energy to socialise instead. You can also find ways to deal with emotional triggers. Before reaching for a snack, ask yourself, 'Am I hungry for food or hungry for stress-release, love or attention?' If it's the latter, build love, laughter and balance into your daily life.

Finally, don't worry if you feel you need to treat yourself every now and again. An occasional sweet, cake, chocolate or piece of fresh white bread won't hurt. Sometimes these things can cheer you up. A glass of wine or two may be just what you fancy. So go ahead and enjoy it. Remember, everything is good in moderation; just don't get into the habit of turning to alcohol as the only way to relax. The same applies to tea, coffee and chocolate: as long as you're eating the good stuff daily, it really isn't terrible if you eat the bad stuff once in a while. However, if you're eating it regularly because you often have bad days, you need to rethink your life as well as your diet.

Midlife eating disorders

We usually think of eating disorders – such as anorexia, bulimia and binge eating – as the territory of teenage girls. In recent years, however, more and more midlife women have developed similar problems. Research shows that these unhealthy eating-related behaviours are driven not so much by concern about appearance as they tend to be in younger women but by depression, anxiety, perfectionism, menopausal symptoms and, especially, dieting.

That's right – diets, even short ones. Why? Because we start them with the mindset that we're going to stay on them until we reach a certain goal and then come off them again. This on-again, off-again diet mentality encourages obsessions, ratchets up anxiety and depression, triggers bingeing and ensures failure.

The solution, then, is not to go on another diet. Instead, you'll need to learn to think about food, weight, your body and yourself in brand new ways. That's because eating disorders begin with a thought, usually an errant one, such as, 'If I can just lose 20 pounds, my life will be great' or 'I can't control myself around food' or 'Now that I've blown it, I might as well eat whatever I want for the rest of the day'.

Why does this happen? It happens because today's midlife woman is typically under tremendous stress as she struggles to raise children, work full-time, take care of ailing parents, hold a relationship together and deal with the physical signs of ageing. Many women turn to unhealthy eating-related behaviours to ease anxiety and tension, and to avoid facing some of life's more difficult problems. So, for example, a woman may go on a strict diet to lose 20 pounds in an attempt to revive a failing marriage.

Disordered eating patterns can also be a way of coping with life in general. If your life is in upheaval, sticking to a very restrictive diet may give you a sense of control. If you're anxious or depressed, bingeing may be a way to comfort yourself. If your emotions are bottled up, purging can be a way to express anger and frustration.

Fortunately, midlife eating disorders can be treated. By identifying and replacing the unhealthy thoughts that bring on unhealthy behaviours, you can – with the support of a doctor or counsellor – regain control of your eating behaviours. Then, by eating healthy, regular meals and learning to alleviate the anxiety, depression and perfectionism that fuel disordered eating, you can re-establish a healthy relationship with food and your own body.

If you have developed an unhealthy relationship with food it's important that you get help and support to reduce the serious health risks associated with a poor diet. Your doctor can put you in touch with a dietitian or help you find a counsellor or cognitive behavioural therapist who specialises in eating problems. If you prefer to go it alone, you can also get support from eating disorder organisations and specialist centres.

How to curb your appetite and eat less

Learning how to curb your appetite is a powerful way to stress-proof your diet and help you lose weight. The Menopause Diet and detox guidelines – in particular the eating little and often strategy (*see page 30*) – will help you beat food cravings. However, you can also use some psychological, emotional and common-sense strategies to completely change your approach to eating. These strategies can help regulate your appetite effectively and efficiently for the rest of your life.

We know that doing things like food shopping when we're hungry is a bad idea as it makes us far more likely to binge on calorie-rich, sugary, fatty foods. So here are some less obvious strategies that can help you control your appetite rather than letting it control you.

Take time over your meals

This strategy seems simple but is harder than you think. These days, eating on the go or grabbing a snack has become commonplace, but if you take time over your meals, really chew your food and taste what you're eating, you're less likely to over eat. Try it for yourself and you'll see that it works. Put your knife and fork down after each mouthful and chew your food slowly. If you think you need to eat more, wait 10 or 15 minutes to see if you're still hungry. Your brain lags behind your stomach by about 20 minutes when it comes to satiety (fullness) signals. If you eat slowly enough, your brain will catch up to tell you that you're no longer in need of dessert.

Take time over your shopping and cooking too, and make eating an occasion. Never eat while standing up or on the go. Sit down for your meals, switch off the television and radio and take your time. Enjoy conversation with your loved ones while you eat, and if you live alone listen to some soothing music. If you never have time to cook or sit down for a meal it really is time to rethink your priorities. You are what you eat. If you take the time to think about what you eat and eat well you will have more physical and mental energy. You'll look and feel better and cope more easily with life's challenges. What could be more important?

Get a good night's sleep

A good night's sleep is important as a lack of sleep disrupts hormones, triggering changes in your metabolism so you don't process food as well as you could. It's thought that lack of sleep is linked with higher levels of cortisol which can throw the metabolism out of balance. Other studies have shown that sleep deprivation can have a negative effect on carbohydrate metabolism and endocrine function, lowering glucose tolerance. This makes it more difficult to convert carbohydrates into energy, and easier for fats and sugars to be stored as unwanted extra pounds.

Other research has established a link between lack of sleep and increased appetite, largely because cortisol is important in appetite control. Researchers at Columbia University Medical Center in New York found that people with low levels of the hormone leptin have trouble maintaining weight loss after dieting. Leptin is produced during sleep, suggesting that shift workers and others with abnormal sleeping patterns may face a higher risk of obesity. (*For some tips on getting a good night's sleep, see Chapter 8, page 182.*)

Don't eat dinner late

Try to finish dinner no later than 8pm. In the evening your body's metabolism naturally slows down, and dinner time is when your body needs the smallest meal. If you get home late, skip dinner. Have a light snack instead, such as a bowl of soup or some low-fat yoghurt and fruit.

Studies have found that the more you eat in the morning, the less you'll eat in the evening. You also have more opportunity to burn off those early-day calories.

Choose your eating spot

It's important that you designate a spot where you eat, such as at your kitchen or dining table. If you learn to always sit down at the same place, research shows you are less likely to graze on the go. Psychologically, you come to associate eating when at home with that place only.

Once you've designated your eating spot, make sure your table and chair are in the warmest part of that room. Perhaps the sun shines on a particular spot, or maybe during the winter you can sit next to the radiator. Research shows that the hotter we feel, the more our appetite is switched off.

Don't sit comfortably. It's important to select a dining chair that isn't too comfortable. That way you'll spend less time sitting and eating, and you'll be less tempted to serve yourself a second portion. Obviously if you have family members or guests to eat, they should have normal dining chairs – but not you.

Whether you eat in your kitchen or dining room, paint it in a shade you wouldn't normally choose. Research has shown that rooms that are welcoming in their colours and decor make people feel like spending longer relaxing in them. Spending longer in the kitchen or dining room equals more grazing.

Choose your plate carefully

Research has shown that eating from plates that are a shade of mid-blue actually switches off your appetite. Also, put away dinner-size plates and eat off salad-size ones instead. Smaller plates play a visual trick on you, giving you a sense that you're eating a bigger portion. Your eyes become used to a smaller plate and portion size rather than wanting to fill up on bigger portions.

Change your habits

Small changes can result in big weight loss. Focus on a typical week and think of three things you could do differently to help you lose weight. For example, swap a large latte for a regular; eat a handful of crisps instead of the whole bag; have a handful of nuts instead of bread before a meal.

Drink up

Drinking a glass of water before you eat can aid weight loss because you feel fuller. Water helps to flush out toxins and waste but it's also very important for weight loss as fat can be broken down only when water is present. Water can also have a direct impact on energy – we may reach for a sugar fix when what we really need is to rehydrate the body.

Drinking four cups of green tea each day is said to help you lose weight. Studies at the American Society for Clinical Nutrition found that one of the compounds in green tea – catechol – increases metabolism and reduces the amount of fat your body absorbs by as much as 30 per cent. Green tea is rich in natural antioxidants that fight the damaging effects of free radicals. They include vitamin B5, which plays a key role in the body's metabolism, and vitamins B1 and B2, which are essential for releasing energy from food.

Eat soup

Having a bowl of soup may help you lose weight. Researchers at Johns Hopkins University in Baltimore, USA, found that people who chose soup as a starter consumed 25 per cent less fat in the following main meal than those who chose a high-fat starter.

Get minted

Having something minty between meals or while eating, such as green tea, has been shown to switch off appetite. Another idea if you feel like snacking when you aren't hungry but bored is to brush your teeth with a minty toothpaste, again to help switch off your appetite. And to stave off cravings for a post-meal sweet, finish a meal with mint tea, a peppermint or even some chewing gum.

Tune in

Before resorting to a comforting snack, reach for your CD player or iPod and play your favourite mood-boosting music. Simply listening to a few minutes of upbeat music has been shown to distract people from hunger pangs. Going for a walk can have a similar effect.

Become a pin-up

Pin up a photograph of you from a time when you were happy and a healthy weight. The fridge door is the best place because each time you open it you'll think about the size and shape you know you can be. This is a reminder not to raid it. If the biscuit tin is your worst enemy then stick your photo on top of it.

Phone a friend

Sometimes you may need a helping hand to control your appetite. You can enlist the support of a friend as a crisis buddy so it's agreed that you'll ring them when you're about to comfort eat. Or you can simply call when you're tempted to reach for food you don't really need. Engaging in pleasant conversation has been shown to soothe frayed nerves that may otherwise lead to overeating.

Stroke a pet or hug a loved one

This has been shown to be comforting, and people who feel comforted and loved are less likely to snack. So use stroking your pet or hugging someone you care about to soothe away the temptation to eat when you don't really need to.

Sniff a banana, apple or peppermint

You might feel silly, but it works. When Alan R. Hirsch, MD, neurological director of the Smell & Taste Treatment and Research Foundation in Chicago, tried this with 3,000 volunteers, he found that the more frequently people sniffed, the less hungry they were and the more weight they lost – an average of 30 pounds each. One theory is that sniffing the food tricks the brain into thinking you're actually eating it.

Why not have a go with cocoa butter hand lotion? When you get a craving for chocolate or sweets, sniff your hand cream as you rub it in. It kills two birds with one stone, leading to softer skin and less snacking. Stimulating your senses with a delicious scent, such as vanilla or mint, has been shown to switch off cravings. You don't need to invest in expensive scent patches.

Try acupuncture

Properly applied, acupuncture removes hunger pangs by stimulating the release of the so-called pleasure hormones, endorphins, which are stimulated by food. Because acupuncture does the work of food in this way, your stomach doesn't miss it and hunger pangs don't occur. Moreover, specialists in acupuncture claim that the effects last even after the course of acupuncture is over.

Serve your dinner restaurant style
Try serving food on plates, restaurant style, rather than in family-style bowls and platters. When your plate is empty, you've finished, and there's no reaching for seconds.

Look in the mirror
Hang a mirror opposite your seat at the table. One study found that eating in front of mirrors slashed the amount people ate by nearly a third. It seems that having to look yourself in the eye reflects back some of your inner standards and goals, and reminds you why you're trying to lose weight in the first place.

Put out a vegetable platter
Research from Pennsylvania State University found that eating water-rich foods such as courgettes, tomatoes and cucumbers during meals reduces overall calorie consumption. Other water-rich foods include soups and salads.

Use vegetables to bulk up meals. You can eat twice as much pasta salad loaded with veggies like broccoli, carrots and tomatoes for the same calories as a pasta salad sporting just mayonnaise. The same goes for stir-fries.

Switch to ordinary coffee
Fancy coffee drinks from trendy coffee bars often pack several hundred calories thanks to whole milk, whipped cream, sugar and syrups. A cup of ordinary coffee with skimmed milk has just a fraction of those calories. And when brewed with good beans, it tastes just as great.

Eat cereal for breakfast

Studies have found that people who eat cereal for breakfast every day are significantly less likely to be obese and have diabetes than those who don't. They also consume more fibre and calcium and less fat than those who eat other breakfast foods. Of course, that doesn't mean reaching for the Coco Pops. Instead, pour out a high-fibre, low-sugar cereal like oat porridge.

Eat most of your meals at home

You're more likely to eat more – and eat more high-fat, high-calorie foods – when you eat out than when you eat at home. Restaurants today serve such large portions that many have switched to larger plates and tables to accommodate them!

Walk up and down some stairs

Whenever you're hungry, walk up and down the stairs. Doing this for just 10 minutes a day could help you shed as much as 10 pounds a year (assuming you're eating healthily as well), according to the Centre for Disease Control.

Take a walk before dinner

You'll do more than burn calories – you'll cut your appetite. In a study of 10 obese women conducted at the University of Glasgow, 20 minutes of walking reduced appetite and increased sensations of fullness as effectively as a light meal.

Get cleaning

Once a week, wash something thoroughly, such as a floor, a couple of windows, the shower cubicle, bathroom tiles or your car. A 150-pound person who dons rubber gloves and exerts some elbow grease will burn about four calories for every minute spent cleaning. Scrub for 30 minutes and you could work off approximately 120 calories, the same number in half a cup/4oz of vanilla frozen yoghurt.

Snack on almonds

Substitute a handful of almonds for a sugary snack. A study from the City of Hope National Medical Center found that overweight people who ate a moderate-fat diet containing almonds lost more weight than a control group that didn't eat nuts.

Make one social outing a week an active one

Pass on the movie tickets and screen the views of a local park instead. Not only will you sit less, but you'll be saving calories too by not eating that bucket of popcorn. You could also plan a tennis match, sign up for a guided nature or city walk (check your local newspaper), go cycling on a bike path or join a sports team.

Watch one hour less of television

A study of 76 undergraduate students found the more they watched television, the more often they ate and the more they ate overall. Sacrifice one programme and go for a walk instead. You'll have time left over to finish a chore or spend some quality time with your loved ones.

Order your dressing on the side

Stick a fork in it – your dressing, not your salad. The small amount of dressing that clings to the tines of the fork is plenty for the forkful of salad you then pick up.

Order wine by the glass, not the bottle
That way you'll be more aware of how much alcohol you're downing. Moderate drinking can be good for your health, but alcohol is high in calories.

Kiss

Passionately kiss your partner 10 times a day. According to the 1991 *Kinsey Institute New Report on Sex*, a passionate kiss burns 6.4 calories per minute. Ten minutes a day of kissing equates to about 23,000 calories – or eight pounds – a year!

Things you never knew could make you gain weight

Hay fever or allergies
Many allergy sufferers find that antihistamines increase their appetite. Not only that, but those with hay fever can also wake up hundreds of times each night, a problem known as 'microarousal', leaving them feeling exhausted and more likely to reach for comfort foods for energy.

E-mail
Are you guilty of e-mailing your colleagues instead of walking over to speak to them face to face? If so, you're likely to gain a pound a year.

Artificial sweeteners
There's some evidence suggesting that artificial sweeteners can play tricks on your body's natural ability to monitor its calorie intake, so be mindful of that if you find yourself using a lot of artificial sweetener. Everything in moderation!

Also, drinks high in fructose can suppress appetite-regulating chemicals in our bodies. So you're better off eating whole fruit and opting for herbal teas.

Too much low fat

A lot of so-called low-fat and fat-free foods offer reduced carbs and fat, but they are often high in sugar and calories and low in nutrients. The exceptions are low-fat yoghurt, cheese and milk, which provide some important nutrients.

Anxiety

Chronic stress increases levels of the hormone cortisol. Elevated cortisol is associated with insulin resistance and increased abdominal fat – a great reason to book that relaxing massage!

Skipping meals

Every time you eat, your metabolic rate speeds up by 20–30 per cent for the next two hours, but if you skip meals you miss out on this. Missing breakfast is the biggest problem – your metabolic rate slows by 5 per cent overnight and stays at this rate until you next eat.

Toxic overload

Are you taking care of your liver? The liver is the main fat-burning organ of the body, but if it's overloaded with toxins such as alcohol, it's too busy handling these to process fat effectively. So cut down on the booze, refined sugar and saturated fat.

Fast-food salads
Fast-food salads can contain more calories than a burger. A McDonald's Chicken Caesar Salad with dressing has 452 calories compared to 375 in a McChicken Sandwich. If you want to eat fast food now and again it pays to do your research.

Your birthday
It's been suggested that babies born in winter are more prone to obesity than those born in summer. The reasoning behind this is a little fuzzy and inconclusive, but one idea is that winter babies have slower metabolic rates.

Watching television
If this doesn't get you away from the box, nothing will. Experts at Tulane University in the US have discovered that heart rate, blood pressure and metabolic rate slow so much while we watch television that we burn 20–30 fewer calories an hour than if we simply sat still.

Brown bread
Be warned: most brown bread is as refined as white bread. Choose granary, wholegrain or seeded breads because they take longer for the body to digest and don't trigger insulin surges.

Your taste buds
People with relatively few taste buds tend to consume foods high in sugar and fat, because it's our taste buds that tell us how much of these foods we've eaten. If this sounds like you, cut down on the foods that make you want more!

Too many late nights

Fatigue interferes with our ability to process carbs and slows down the metabolic rate, so make sure you get to bed at a reasonable hour.

Thyroid trouble and PCOS

Thyroid dysfunction can cause a lower metabolic rate and make it very difficult to lose weight. If you're tired all the time, gaining weight and really feeling the cold, then your thyroid could be sluggish, which in turn slows down your metabolism. Combat it by consulting your doctor for advice. You might also want to ask your doctor to rule out PCOS or polycystic ovaries, which can cause problems with weight loss. Common symptoms of PCOS include irregular periods, excess body hair, acne and weight gain.

Moving in together

When you're deeply in love, the last thing you're likely to be thinking about is your waistline. Nor should you, but sharing every little thing equally is not always the way to go. One case in point is portion sizes. Just because you now live together doesn't mean you have to match him bite for bite.

Have the Right Mindset

Think long-term lifestyle change instead of short-term fix and your chances of success with weight loss are high. Also, don't think you have to rely on the scales to set a goal; find other ways to measure your success such as a dress size down or improvements in your energy levels. If you do pick a number on the scales, give yourself a 5 pound weight-range target as it's not realistic to maintain a constant weight.

Studies show that a positive, optimistic attitude about your ability to lose weight increases your chances of success. The right mindset also means being comfortable with slow and gradual weight loss. If you're losing more than two pounds a week, the chances are you're losing muscle and water, and the more muscle you lose the slower you will burn calories.

Above all, try not to get stressed about losing weight. Instead, use your energy to motivate you to eat healthily and exercise regularly, not just for a few weeks but for the rest of your life. If you follow the Menopause Diet and detox guidelines and are focused on feeling fit and healthy, natural weight loss – along with a reduction in symptoms as you approach menopause – will follow.

All about Supplements

If you're following the Menopause Diet guidelines you should be getting all the nutrients you need to balance your hormones and lose weight. However, because certain nutrients are essential during menopause, taking supplements may be extremely helpful.

As we age we absorb less of the nutrients we once did. To protect your heart, bones and health in the years approaching menopause you can't afford to be deficient in any nutrients. Therefore, on top of your Menopause Diet and lifestyle detox, it might be wise to take a daily multivitamin and mineral supplement containing:

- vitamins A, D, E, C, B1, B2, B3, B5, B6, B13
- folic acid
- calcium
- magnesium
- iron
- zinc
- chromium
- selenium
- manganese
- boron

You may need to take two or more tablets a day to meet your requirements. Vitamin C, calcium and magnesium are bulky so may need to be taken separately.

Bear in mind that even though supplements are a good insurance policy they should never replace healthy eating because they can't offer the same beneficial effects. Food contains a variety of different elements such as fibre, water and nutrients that simply can't appear in dried capsules or powders.

Nutritional Supplements

A good quality multivitamin and mineral should form the foundation of your supplement programme to make sure you have adequate nutrients for hormone balance and healthy bones. If you feel you need an extra helping hand, you can add other supplements that have suggested positive results in connection with menopause. (For supplement recommendations for specific symptoms of menopause, *see Chapter 8.*)

Make sure you buy supplements from reputable companies that focus on quality control and, if you so request, can supply an independent analysis of their products. You should take your multivitamin and mineral every day from now on but this won't necessarily apply to all the supplements listed below. For best results take them for the short term, say a period of three to four months. After that reassess them for improvements in your health and adjust your supplement programme accordingly.

WARNING

Certain supplements, such as vitamin A, can be toxic in large doses so it's important to consult a nutritionist, pharmacist and/or doctor to ensure the dosages are correct. If you're on any kind of medication, have high blood pressure, insulin resistance or are pregnant or hoping to be, consult your doctor before taking supplements of any kind. If you're considering herbal medicine make sure you discuss it with your doctor and consult a trained herbalist first.

Supplements A to Z

Antioxidants

If you're eating a healthy diet and taking a multivitamin and mineral supplement you may not need to take additional antioxidants unless advised by your doctor or nutritional therapist. Antioxidants are abundant in fruits, vegetables and sprouted grains so make sure you get plenty of these foods in your diet. If, however, you exercise a lot or are exposed to a great deal of stress or chemical pollutants, it might be wise to add an antioxidant complex to your supplement programme.

Boron

A study published in the *British Journal of Nutrition* in 1993 showed that increasing dietary intake of the mineral boron from 0.25mg daily to 3.25mg raised levels of oestradiol (a form of oestrogen) in post-menopausal women while decreasing the amount of calcium excreted in the urine. That means less risk of bone loss. Studies by the Department of Agriculture in the US found similar benefits for a high-boron diet (3mg per day). Make sure your multivitamin and mineral supplement contains enough boron. There are 2mg of boron in 100g (3½oz) of almonds, prunes or raisins. Asparagus, cabbage, figs, peaches and strawberries are good sources as well.

B vitamin complex

B vitamins are incredibly helpful during times of stress. Symptoms of B vitamin deficiency include anxiety, tension, irritability and poor concentration. If this sounds familiar or if you're under a great deal of stress it might be a good idea to supplement with additional B vitamins for a few months to get your health and energy back. You should be getting about

50mg of most of the B vitamins a day, so if your multivitamin isn't giving you enough add a B complex to your supplement plan.

Calcium

This mineral helps guard against osteoporosis. Calcium also appears to improve blood sugar balance, and recent studies have shown that extra calcium can help with weight loss. The UK's National Academy of Sciences considers 1,000mg of calcium a day adequate for women between 31 and 50, and 1,200mg a day adequate for women of 51 and over. Most experts agree that you should try to get all the calcium you can through diet, but some women – particularly vegans – may need to supplement to reach those levels. If this applies to you, talk to your doctor about using a calcium supplement. Good sources of calcium include low-fat dairy products, brazil nuts, almonds, sesame seeds, salmon with bones and green leafy vegetables.

C vitamin

Vitamin C is a powerful immune booster but is particularly helpful at menopause. Giving women vitamin C with bioflavonoids has been shown to reduce hot flushes. Vitamin C helps to build up collagen. This gives your skin and tissues elasticity and can therefore be useful in the treatment of vaginal dryness and stress incontinence. Collagen is also important for strong bones. Vitamin C is abundant in fruits and vegetables but you may also want to supplement your diet with 1,000mg per day of vitamin C and bioflavonoids.

D vitamin

This vitamin helps with the absorption of calcium. Dietary intake of vitamin D has decreased over recent years and may be linked to rising cases of osteoporosis. Vitamin D supplements can be toxic in high doses so it's best to make sure your multivitamin and mineral contains vitamin D and to get plenty of exposure to daylight. Fatty fish, such as halibut, mackerel and salmon, is a rich source of vitamin D. Other sources include low-fat dairy products and fortified cereals.

Essential fatty acids (EFAs)

Dry skin, cracked nails, lifeless hair, depression, aching joints, lack of energy, weight-management problems, forgetfulness, vaginal dryness and breast pain are all symptoms of menopause and deficiency in essential fatty acids. Components of these fatty acids may protect you from heart disease because they're believed to increase 'good' HDL cholesterol while lowering triglyceride levels and blood pressure – that's why supplementing with EFAs during menopause can help with many symptoms. In addition to making sure your diet is rich in EFAs from oily fish, nuts and seeds, take 1–2 tablespoons of a cold-pressed blend of fish oils providing omega 3 essential fats. If you're a vegetarian and prefer not to take fish oil then flaxseed/linseed or hempseed oil is fine.

E vitamin

Although clinical trials have produced unimpressive results, this heart protector is thought to be a good bet for the relief of hot flushes, breast tenderness and vaginal dryness. It's used topically for vaginal dryness, and there may be benefits from taking it orally as well. The recommended daily allowance (RDA) for vitamin E is 15mg (22IU) but some experts recommend a therapeutic dose of 400IU, and getting this amount daily from food isn't easy. Asparagus, avocados, brown rice, egg yolks, lima beans, peas, sweet potatoes and vegetable oils (like corn and soya) are the best food sources. If you have a bleeding disorder or diabetes, or take blood thinning medication, check with your doctor before supplementing with vitamin E.

Magnesium

This mineral has a calming effect, easing symptoms like irritability, anxiety, mood swings and insomnia. It also helps your bones absorb calcium, raises levels of 'good' HDL cholesterol while lowering 'bad' LDL cholesterol, and helps muscles – including your heart – to relax.

The standard recommended amount for adult women is 320mg a day. Good sources are almonds, cashews, escarole, kale, kelp and wheat bran. For example, 30g (1oz) of almonds give you 77mg of magnesium.

How Can I Tell if I'm Deficient in a Particular Nutrient?

Although serious nutritional deficiencies are easy to spot (lack of vitamin C causes gums to bleed, for example), low intakes aren't so easy to detect. Hair and mineral analysis isn't always easy. A quick way to determine if you need to take supplements is to check out the website of the Health Supplements Information Service at www.hsis.org. Use the nutrition calculator devised by Dr Ann Walker to check your intake from specific food groups and to give you an idea of the supplements you might benefit from taking.

Controlling Symptoms the Natural Way

Natural herbal supplements to treat menopause symptoms have been on the rise because they tend to work gently without severe side-effects. Many women have found relief from their menopause symptoms by using them. The main herbs are called adaptogens. If you have a low level of one hormone or an excess of another, the herb will have a balancing effect on your hormones and your body.

> **WARNING**
>
> As long as you discuss your choice of nutritional supplements with your doctor, they are fine to take alongside HRT, but this doesn't apply to the herbs and natural therapies listed below. Using herbs in combination with HRT could overload your body with oestrogen. Quite simply, if you're taking HRT you shouldn't need to take herbs to ease your symptoms. If you're still having hot flushes and other symptoms you need to speak to your GP.

Agnus castus

This is one of the most important herbs you can take at menopause because it works as an adaptogen, helping to balance your hormones. It appears to stimulate and normalise the function of the pituitary gland, which controls and regulates the hormones in the body, and is a potent remedy for hot flushes. Available from health food stores, herbalists and nutritional therapists, agnus castus is usually marketed under the name Vitex. It should be taken for a period of several months to determine efficacy. Side-effects include digestive upsets and a mild rash. A typical recommended dose of Vitex organic tincture is one teaspoon three times a day for three or four months. The herb can be taken daily for up to 18 continuous months.

Before taking Vitex, check with your doctor that it's safe for you to do so. If depression is one of your symptoms you should probably avoid agnus castus as some research suggests that depression may be related to excess progesterone, and agnus castus can raise progesterone levels.

Black cohosh

This herbal remedy has been used for centuries to help alleviate menopause symptoms, especially hot flushes and vaginal dryness. Many experts believe its effectiveness lies in its ability to diminish the levels of luteinizing hormone, which is manufactured by the body in elevated amounts during menopause. Although popular, black cohosh isn't recommended here because there have been recent reports of toxic effects on the liver with long-term use.

Dong quai

This Chinese herb is widely available in Western health food stores. It's similar to agnus castus (*see above*) and can be used for long periods of time because it's a tonic herb. It nourishes the liver and is said to help ease menopausal symptoms, such as hot flushes and vaginal dryness, although research has yet to prove this conclusively. It's widely used among Chinese women because of its reputation as a libido and energy booster, and has been dubbed the 'female ginseng'.

Evening primrose oil

Evening primrose oil is most commonly used for relieving premenstrual syndrome, tender breasts and menopausal symptoms. It's rich in GLA and linolenic acid – essential fats the body requires to regulate hormones. Evening primrose oil is prescribed in the UK under the brand name Efamest. The dose recommended by doctors is around 1,000mg per day, but most experts agree that although it can improve skin quality and soothe tender breasts, it has little benefit for hot flushes.

Natural progesterone cream/wild yam

Natural progesterone is thought to offset oestrogen dominance, one of the most common conditions in perimenopause and the underlying cause of a host of symptoms (*see Chapter 1, page 11*). Unlike synthetic progesterone manufactured in a lab, natural progesterone is made from a substance found in wild yams and soya beans. The progesterone it produces is almost identical to that produced by the body. Although many women have found relief from the symptoms of menopause with natural progesterone creams there are downsides as well, and some women end up feeling worse.

Natural progesterone comes in several forms including capsule, topical cream to rub on your skin, vaginal suppository and sublingual drops to place under the tongue. You won't be able to get it over the counter as it's available only on prescription. Many experts recommend the topical cream rather than the capsules because the cream is easily absorbed and gradually released into the body in a similar way to the ovaries' natural release of progesterone.

Wild yam extracts are sometimes confused with natural progesterone. This is because natural progesterone is synthesised from the chemical compound diosgenin, found in soya beans and wild yam. There have been suggestions, therefore, that the use of wild yam cream (which contains diosgenin) will increase progesterone levels. This is incorrect, as the human body doesn't have the enzymes capable of converting diosgenin into progesterone. Similarly, any cream sold over the counter (not obtained on prescription) claiming to contain natural progesterone is fraudulent. It's safer and more effective to get a prescription for a natural progesterone cream from your doctor.

Isoflavones

Isoflavones derived from soy are another popular natural menopause remedy. They contain phytoestrogens, which some experts speculate are able to mimic the function of the female hormone oestrogen, thereby possibly reducing hot flushes and some other menopause symptoms.

Soya isoflavones should be a strong consideration to include in your Menopause Diet, through either food or drink sources. As far as supplements are concerned, the recommended dose is 40–80mg a day – the same dose used in some studies for the treatment of hot flushes – but it can take several weeks before beneficial effects are seen. The long-term effects of these fairly new supplements are as yet unknown, so if you decide to take isoflavone supplements – perhaps in the form of red clover – it might be better to do so for a short period only while you work on including more phytoestrogens in your diet (*see Chapter 3, page 47*).

Milk thistle

Milk thistle can be an important herb at menopause because it helps boost liver function and makes sure old hormones are being excreted efficiently. Up to three 500mg tablets or capsules daily can help you detox gently.

Valerian

This herb has been used for thousands of years to ease insomnia and improve sleep quality. If the herbs and supplements here aren't making much of a difference to your symptoms, you could consider using valerian.

Suggested Supplement Plan

- A good multivitamin and mineral supplement (*see page 139*).
- Flaxseed/linseed oil (1,000mg per day).
- A mixture of equal parts of agnus castus, dong quai and milk thistle. Take one teaspoon two or three times a day. If you have problems getting to sleep, try valerian. Take herbs for three or four months, and if symptoms don't improve consult your GP.
- Nutritional supplements specifically designed for menopause: stick to reputable companies, such as Boots, that can back up their products with research. Menopace is the only menopause supplement endorsed by BUPA. It's been specifically designed to provide a comprehensive amount of vitamins, minerals and nutrients to balance your hormones (*see www.menopace.com*).

Menopause SOS

Following the Menopause Diet and doing the gentle Detox Boost will greatly increase your chances of sailing through the menopause with few, if any, symptoms. You may, however, have a specific symptom or condition that's a cause of concern for you. This chapter provides advice to help you beat the most common symptoms of menopause and reduce the three most common health risks.

The symptoms listed here are all related to a drop in oestrogen. The list may seem daunting, but fortunately no woman experiences the whole range – you'll probably experience only a few symptoms, and some women have none at all.

For a list of the food sources of essential nutrients mentioned in this chapter, refer to the Essential Nutrients Guide (*page 225*). For more information about specific supplements, refer to Chapter 7.

WARNING

If at any point your symptoms become unmanageable, consult your doctor immediately. If you want to try herbal remedies make sure you discuss this with your doctor first and talk to a trained herbalist to ensure there are no contraindications. Avoid herbal therapies altogether if you are taking medication or have a pre-existing medical condition.

A to Z of the Most Common Symptoms of Menopause and Natural Ways to Treat Them

Aches and pains

Aching joints and muscle problems are common before, during and after menopause. The joint pain isn't caused by injury or exhaustion but may be related to fluctuating hormone levels. Collagen is a protein that binds every tissue in the body. When it begins to weaken at menopause, muscles lose their bulk, strength and coordination, and joints become stiff. Muscles become more prone to stiffness after exercise and joints may swell so movement is restricted. If you experience bloating and fluid retention you may also get pins and needles or numbness in your hands.

It isn't wise to ignore aches and pains as early treatment can often bring about a cure and prevent further development of arthritis. Getting plenty of rest, eating nutritious foods – preferably organic, especially fruits and vegetables – and avoiding known toxins and stimulants are healthy strategies for fighting joint pains. The following recommendations should also help:

- Try a heating pad or soaking in a warm bath for 30 minutes to increase the blood flow to the muscles. Try adding a valerian essential oil to the bath water. A warm footbath with a few drops of peppermint or rosemary essential oil just before bed may help. Ginger baths, soaks and compresses may bring soothing, warm relief to sore and aching joints.
- Try to exercise every day. If you're in a lot of pain avoid high-impact exercises and do yoga, stretching and walking instead.
- Avoid over-the-counter painkillers unless absolutely necessary. Capsaicin creams may prove useful if applied several times a day. Other herbal remedies that may be

helpful include alfalfa, feverfew and white willow. Unlike aspirin and cortisone, these herbs don't produce side-effects when used carefully. Also unlike drugs, herbs provide bone-building minerals, immune-strengthening micronutrients and endocrine-nourishing glycosides. Salicylates found in the bark, buds and leaves of willows, birches, true wintergreen, poplars and black haw have been used for centuries to help ease inflammatory pain. Sterols found in the roots of many plants such as wild yam, sarsaparilla, ginseng and devil's club have also been found to help ease sore joints.

- Blackcurrant bud macerate is an anti-inflammatory that may be a wonderful ally for post-menopausal women with arthritis, rheumatism, allergies, headaches and persistent hot flushes. A 30–50 drop dose may be used up to three times a day.
- Essential fatty acids have anti-inflammatory properties. A spoonful of fresh flaxseed/linseed or evening primrose oil several times a day may relieve pain within a few days, and regular use helps prevent aching joints.
- In addition to herbal remedies, visualisation, swimming in warm water and acupuncture may greatly help aching joints.
- Pay attention to your posture including how you sit, stand or carry items, and try to reduce the strain on your back and neck. When standing, keep your head held high, your pelvis forward and your abdomen and buttocks tucked in. When sitting, keep your spine against the back of the chair and your knees a little higher than your hips. When carrying items, remember that heavy bags put pressure on your back so try to alter the load.
- If you have regular severe back and neck pain that doesn't come and go with your menstrual cycle, consult your doctor for recommendations and back-strengthening exercises.

Acne

You might have thought you'd left breakouts behind with teenage angst, and then suddenly your skin starts to erupt again. Falling oestrogen levels are to blame, changing your body's balance to testosterone. Stress can also be a trigger. You may notice that your spots cluster around the lower part of your face. They may appear as angry red lumps rather than popable pimples, and since adult pimples are darker than teen ones, the ensuing discolouration can last a few weeks.

Prescription drugs should be your last resort as they won't address the real cause of the problem. Try to identify the trigger factor. If it's stress, aim for eight hours' sleep a night and take time out each day for meditation, yoga or other forms of relaxation. Although there's no known cure for acne, the following remedies may help keep the blemishes under control:

- It's important to include plenty of phytoestrogens in your diet (*see Chapter 3*). Phytoestrogens can help your body control the amount of testosterone circulating in your blood. Vitamin B6, zinc and essential fatty acids have also been shown to be beneficial.
- While there's no known relationship between specific foods and acne flare-ups, if you notice any dietary triggers for acne, avoid these foods. You should also watch your intake of alcohol, sugar, processed food, salt, butter, caffeine, chocolate, fried foods, meat, margarine, wheat, soft drinks and foods containing hydrogenated vegetable oils.
- To ease inflammation or prevent infection, eat lots of garlic. Garlic is a powerful antibiotic. Grate it on your food or take it as a supplement every day.
- Sulphur-rich foods such as eggs and onion, and live yoghurt with bifidus and acidophilus bacteria, help to rebalance the bacteria in your gut and can help protect against skin inflammation.

- Regular exercise is helpful because it encourages hormonal balance and healthy blood flow to your face to help flush out toxins.
- Heavy cosmetics and rich moisturisers can clog your pores so use a lighter lotion on your trouble zones. Avoid abrasive scrubs. Although they remove dead skin, they can cause infection and make acne worse. Use one specifically recommended by a dermatologist if you use one at all. Never pick or squeeze spots – this can cause scarring.
- Tea tree oil has good antiseptic, antibacterial and antifungal properties. Use it to dab onto your spots. A study conducted by the Department of Dermatology of the Royal Prince Alfred Hospital in New South Wales, Australia, found a 5 per cent solution of tea tree oil was as effective as a 5 per cent solution of benzoyl peroxide for most cases of acne, and had no side-effects. You may want to use a tea tree moisturiser.
- Pure aloe vera gel is antibacterial and soothing. Some women find that dabbing it on their acne every day really helps. For angry, inflamed spots or acne, witch hazel is cooling and soothing. Dab directly on the acne. Echinacea is one of nature's most powerful antibiotics. Dab a tincture or cream on the affected skin daily.
- If your doctor tells you that you have higher than normal androgen levels, the herb saw palmetto can work as an anti-androgen, and this can be helpful for pre-menstrual acne. Perhaps the most helpful herb, though, is agnus castus. Other beneficial herbs include burdock root, red clover and milk thistle, all of which are powerful blood cleansers. All these remedies should be prescribed by a medical herbalist.
- Light therapy can help. This involves shining different types of light on the acne, from ultraviolet to simple coloured light. Red lights have been shown to open capillaries and boost circulation while blue light closes them. Ask a dermatologist for advice.

Anxiety and irritability

In the run-up to menopause you may feel anxious, trembling or ill at ease and panicky. This is because the parts of your brain that control feelings of wellbeing and contentment are all affected by the absence of oestrogen.

- Take time for yourself when you feel out of control: weeping, yelling, raging and depressed. Create your own special place where you can be alone, without responsibilities. Begin a journal and note your feelings.
- Swings in blood sugar can trigger panic and anxiety so make sure you follow the Menopause Diet guidelines and eat little and often to keep your blood sugar levels and your mood stable.
- It's advisable to avoid tranquillisers, antidepressants, alcohol, cocaine and opium as these drugs may lead to dependence.
- Passionflower helps insomnia and can boost levels of serotonin – the feel-good chemical – in the blood and create a feeling of wellbeing. Passionflower is known to display sedative and analgesic properties, having a calming and restful effect on the central nervous system.
- Motherwort contains alkaloids, tannins and saponins that have antispasmodic and nervine actions, calming the heart and nerves without sedating.
- Valerian root also affects the central nervous system, and has been used in Europe extensively as a sedative and calmative.
- Chamomile (German chamomile) is commonly and successfully used for anxiety and insomnia, in addition to easing indigestion and gastrointestinal inflammations.
- Catnip and peppermint also have a sedative action on the nerves.

- The slow movements and controlled postures of yoga improve muscle strength, flexibility, range of motion, balance, breathing and blood circulation and promote mental focus, clarity and calmness. Stretching also reduces mental and physical stress, tension and anxiety, promotes good sleep, lowers blood pressure and slows down your heart rate.

- Listening to your favourite music is a great method of reducing stress and relieving anxiety. Your preference in music will determine the type of soothing sounds that will best reduce your tension and promote feelings of tranquillity. Pay attention to how you feel when you hear a particular song or genre of music, and keep listening to the ones that produce a relaxing effect.

- Optimism can counteract the negative impact of stress, tension and anxiety on your immune system and wellbeing. Often it's the way you perceive things that determines whether you'll get overwhelmed, both mentally and physically. Having a positive attitude, finding the good in what life throws your way and looking on the bright side enhance your ability to manage stress effectively.

- Relaxing in a hot bath relieves sore muscles and joints, reduces stress and tension, and promotes a good night's sleep. Add some soothing music, soft lighting and naturally scented bath salts or bubble bath to create an inexpensive and convenient spa experience in the privacy of your own home.

- Relaxation techniques such as meditation can promote tranquillity and ease anxiety, and might be worth trying on a regular basis.

Anti-anxiety Foods

Bananas: Women who are depressed or anxious tend to have lower levels of vitamin B6, needed for the production of serotonin, the brain chemical that lifts mood. Low levels of vitamin B12 and folic acid can also cause anxiety. To boost your B vitamins, eat plenty of bananas as well as lean meat and poultry, fish, eggs, nuts, seeds, soya beans and leafy green vegetables.

Whole grains: Women who are deficient in the antioxidant mineral selenium also experience feelings of depression and anxiety. Selenium is found in whole grains as well as meat, fish and shellfish and avocados.

Eggs: Zinc is essential for the body to convert tryptophan into serotonin, the feel-good chemical that can induce feelings of calm. Zinc is found in eggs and also in nuts and seeds, such as peanuts and sunflower seeds.

Oily fish: Not only does eating oily fish reduce your risk of Alzheimer's disease, but according to studies reported in 2003 by the US National Institutes of Health, it reduces anxiety and depression as well.

Nuts and seeds: Foods rich in complex carbohydrates, such as whole grains and legumes, increase brain levels of tryptophan and, in turn, serotonin. A small amount of dietary carbohydrates such as a handful of nuts and seeds, eaten 30 minutes before a stressful situation, can help lower anxiety levels.

Bloating

The hormonal fluctuations that occur during menopause can cause your kidneys to retain water and salt, and this is what makes you feel bloated and heavy. The area under your eyes may also appear puffy, and again this is due to temporary water retention. Over-the-counter remedies are not advised as they can leach valuable nutrients from your body, but if you do get fluid retention there are things you can do to help yourself:

- Cut down on your salt intake. Use less salt in your cooking, watch out for hidden salts in your foods and look for other ways to enhance flavour, such as using herbs and spices instead.
- Increase your fluid intake. You need to drink more, not less, to help your body dilute the salt in your tissues and

allow you to excrete more salt and fluid. Aim to drink at least two to three litres of water a day.

- Reduce the amount of caffeine in your diet. Caffeine is a diuretic, but it won't ease bloating because it hinders the secretion of excess salt and toxins from your body.
- Make sure your diet includes sufficient B vitamins, especially vitamin B6 – found in bananas, lean meat, fish, nuts, seeds and whole grains – which is a tried and tested remedy for water retention.
- Eat foods that naturally decrease fluid retention, like asparagus, apple cider vinegar, alfalfa sprouts and dandelion flowers. Potassium-rich foods will bring down your body's sodium level as the two minerals balance each other out. Reach for those bananas, apricots, black beans, lentils, tomatoes, green leafy vegetables and fresh fruits.
- Keep your blood sugar levels in balance. When levels drop, adrenaline is released to move sugar quickly from your cells into your blood. When the sugar leaves the cells it is replaced by water, which contributes to that bloated feeling.
- Get moving. Moderate exercise will make you sweat and hasten the transport of water through your body.
- Studies at the University of Reading have shown the surprising effectiveness of Colladeen, a mix of grape seed, bilberry and cranberry extract, for relief of bloating.
- Aromatherapy oils can be helpful with bloating. Add fennel or chamomile to a warm bath and soak for 20 minutes for the best effect. You may also want to use juniper as a massage oil.
- Dandelion and parsley are natural herbal diuretics packed with hormone-balancing nutrients that allow fluid to be released without loss of nutrients.
- Elevate your feet if you're prone to swelling in the ankles. Wear supportive stockings to ease discomfort.

- Bloating with abdominal distension may be due to constipation and/or diverticulitis, a condition where small pockets of tissue balloon out from the bowel. In these pockets food may lodge and ferment, producing large pockets of gas. If constipation is the case, refer to the section on digestive problems below. If you suspect diverticulitis – where it's quite common to wake up in the morning with a flat stomach that swells considerably as the day progresses – consult your doctor.

Foods for Beating the Bloat

Olive oil: This promotes the overall absorption of nutrients while helping the digestive system to function more efficiently. It can help reduce bloating because it's very well tolerated by the stomach due to its high oleic acid content. The sphincter, which separates the stomach from the oesophagus, is less affected by olive oil than any other fat – this means less indigestion, acidity and bloating. Two tablespoons of olive oil taken in the morning on an empty stomach also appear to have a positive effect on chronic constipation, another cause of bloating.

Soya yoghurt: Lactobacillus acidophilus is one of the friendly bacteria that live in the intestines. When eaten, it travels to the intestines and crowds out the harmful bacteria that may be causing symptoms of painful gas and bloating. One source of these bacteria is yoghurt that contains live, active culture. It's important to look for yoghurts that specifically say they contain live culture, as many types are heat-treated to kill the bacteria before being sold. For people who either can't tolerate dairy or choose not to eat it, a number of very tasty soya-based yoghurts are available at many health food stores.

Whole grains: These are high in a number of different vitamins and minerals, as well as health-promoting fibre. Fibre prevents constipation, bloating and gas by adding bulk, helping everything move through the intestines more quickly. Whole grains not only relieve the pressure and pain caused by constipation, they also help to feed the friendly bacteria in your gut and therefore protect against gas and bloating. Throughout the day, snack on other high-fibre foods like strawberries, blueberries, dried apricots and dried plums. Be careful not to add too much fibre too quickly or you'll feel even more bloated than before. Your body needs time to get used to processing the increased bulk.

Foods for Beating the Bloat (Cont.)

Bananas: Bloating can also be relieved by vitamin B6, a natural diuretic. Healthy foods that are rich in vitamin B6 include bananas, alfalfa, lentils, oily fish, soya products, raw nuts and seeds (especially walnuts), green leafy vegetables, rye, turkey, oats and brown rice.

Fennel tea: You might also want to try the odd cup of fennel tea. Just brew a tablespoon or so of fennel in a tea strainer and drink several cups a day. Fennel tastes like liquorice and has anti-gas as well as antispasmodic properties, making it especially helpful for bloating. It's also a very safe herbal remedy that you can use daily.

Breast tenderness

Breast swelling and pain, especially in the week or so before your period, are normal reactions to fluctuating hormone levels. As women reach their 40s, however, this discomfort can develop into mastalgia where the breasts become hard and extremely painful. A mastalgia attack can last for up to 10 days. The causes are not completely understood but mastalgia may be due to unusual sensitivity of breast tissue to fluctuating hormones at menopause.

If you experience breast pain, you might fear that it's a symptom of breast cancer. In most cases, mastalgia is a benign condition but you should still see your doctor to have a mammogram and make sure. Then try the recommendations below:

- If you suffer from breast tenderness make sure you wear a comfortable, supportive bra, one that doesn't irritate the nipple area as you move.
- Make sure you get your phytoestrogens, found in foods such as soya, chickpeas and lentils.
- Cut down on foods and drinks containing caffeine. They have been shown to increase problems with tender breasts.

- Up your fibre intake. Research has shown that there may be a link between constipation and a painful breast condition called fibrocystic breast disease. So make sure you drink enough water and have a good intake of fibre to ensure regularity. You may also like to sprinkle some flaxseeds/linseeds on your cereal in the morning. Don't, however, include bran in your diet. Bran can make things worse because it contains substances called phytates, which can interfere with the absorption of important nutrients, like magnesium and calcium.

- Vitamin E has been shown to reduce breast pain and tenderness in some studies. Eat foods rich in vitamin E, such as oats, sunflower oil, whole grains, soya oil and leafy green vegetables. You might also like to take a supplement for a couple of months to give you a kick-start.

- Eat some live yoghurt every day. Breast tenderness may be related to an excess of oestrogen, and the beneficial bacteria in live yoghurt can help to reabsorb old hormones and increase the efficiency of your bowel movements.

- Increase your intake of omega 3 fatty acids. Found in fish oil, these have been shown to relieve breast tenderness and fluid retention. Take fish oil capsules or eat more fish, or sprinkle flaxseeds/linseeds and hemp seeds onto your salads and soups.

- The B vitamins are of particular value if you suffer from breast tenderness because they help your liver break down excess oestrogen. Improve your intake of B vitamin foods and think about taking a B complex supplement for a couple of months.

- Older studies showed that supplementing your diet with evening primrose oil that contains GLA (gamma linoleic acid) could reduce breast discomfort, although more recent studies have not backed this up. The suggested dosage is 240–320mg a day. Do bear in mind, though, that evening primrose oil needs to be taken for about three months to be effective.

- A number of essential oils, such as lavender, fennel and juniper, can encourage lymphatic drainage and help relieve breast pain by regulating hormones. Massage your breasts with them, putting one drop of your chosen oil on a teaspoon of carrier oil such as sweet almond or sunflower, or use a few drops in your bath.
- The herb ginkgo biloba has proved to be effective, according to a French study where women with pre-menstrual breast tenderness taking ginkgo biloba reported less pain than those taking a placebo. Other helpful herbs include agnus castus to balance hormones and milk thistle to help your liver process oestrogen efficiently, allowing excess to be excreted. Ask a medical herbalist for advice.

Breast Self-examination

One of the best ways to protect the health of your breasts is to examine them yourself for lumps at least once a month. Follow the steps below:

1. Lie down and place a pillow under your right shoulder. Next, place your right arm under your head.
2. Using the three middle fingers of your left hand, massage your right breast with the pads of your fingers. Check for any lumps or abnormalities. You can move in a circular motion or up and down. Make sure you use the same motion every month.
3. Continue the motion, extending to the outside of the breast and your armpit.
4. Repeat on the left side.
5. Next, repeat the examination standing up, with one arm behind your shoulder as you examine each breast. Standing or sitting up allows you to feel the outside of the breast more accurately.
6. For an added precaution, stand in front of a mirror and squeeze each nipple. Look for any discharge.
7. Take note of any dimpling, redness or swelling.

Breast Self-examination (Cont.)

If you find anything that concerns you, arrange to see your doctor. The important thing is to learn what is normal for you and to report any changes. These changes may include:

- Any new lump. It may or may not be painful to touch.
- Unusual thick areas.
- Sticky or bloody discharge from your nipples.
- Any changes in the skin of your breasts or nipples, such as puckering or dimpling.
- An unusual increase in the size of one breast.
- One breast unusually lower than the other.

In addition to the examination described above, you may also check your breasts while in the shower. Soapy fingers slide easily across the breast and may increase your chances of detecting a change. While standing in the shower, place one arm over your head and lightly soap your breast on that side. Then, using the flat surface of your fingers – not the fingertips – gently move your hand over your breast, feeling carefully for any lumps or thickened areas.

Depression

Depression or feelings of sadness and apathy may occur during your menopause. This may be caused by centres in your brain that control your state of mind being affected by the absence of oestrogen. Depression is more likely to occur if you are under intense stress and/or there is a family history of depressive illness. If left untreated, depression can be a debilitating illness that can last for years. Consult your doctor if you have experienced four of these symptoms for at least two weeks:

- Unusual sleeping patterns
- Feeling exceptionally apathetic or anxious
- Inability to enjoy things you used to enjoy, including loss of libido
- Extreme fatigue
- Feelings of worthlessness

- Difficulty making simple decisions
- Thoughts of death or suicide (seek help immediately)

Self-help to lift your mood

- If you analyse your thoughts you may be surprised how negative they are. For example, if you drop something you might think, 'Gosh, I'm stupid.' If you bump into someone you might think, 'Why am I so clumsy?' and so on. If you're struggling with your weight you might think, 'I'm fat and ugly.' Try to catch yourself every time you have a negative thought about yourself or the things you do – and counter the thought with one that's more positive or realistic. If you drop something or make a mistake, try: 'Okay, I messed up but what about all the times when I've got things right?' or 'I was looking where I was going and the other person wasn't' and, if you feel very brave, go for 'That wasn't my fault.'
- List all the good things in your life. They could be such things as a job you enjoy, a loyal friend, a fascinating hobby, your dog, the flowers in your garden and so on. Now make a list of all the good things about yourself. Have a good think now as there's bound to be a lot more than you realised. You might be a good listener or a great poet or have a wonderful sense of humour.
- Find new challenges. Taking on a new challenge can be incredibly rewarding and make you feel more positive about yourself. If you've always wanted to learn how to play the piano or keyboard, book some lessons. Consider taking up painting, singing, jewellery making, writing – the list is endless. Perhaps you might like to get some new qualifications or do a course in a subject that might help you deal with your symptoms, such as homeopathy, reflexology, massage and so on.

- Physical activity can contribute to a sense of wellbeing. In fact, regular exercise is considered by some experts to be an effective treatment for depression. Plan to take at least 30 minutes of gentle exercise a day.

- Sing along to your favourite music, have a good cry to release excess stress and a good laugh. Laughter sends chemicals called endorphins whizzing around your body to make you feel naturally high. So do something to get you chuckling, from watching a funny film to calling an old friend.

- St John's wort has been shown in numerous studies to significantly improve depression, anxiety and insomnia. The herb is taken in daily doses of 2–4g, calculated to contain 0.2–1.0mg of the active ingredient hypericin. Capsules containing 300mg of the extract (and 0.3 per cent hypericin) are typically taken three times a day. Consult your doctor if you are considering taking St John's wort to be sure it's safe for you.

- Garden sage, an aromatic member of the mint family, is an ancient ally for depression and emotionally distressed midlife women. It's also said to have mild oestrogenic effects, possibly explaining its use as a hormone-balancing herb that can encourage regular menstruation.

- Ginger has been a powerhouse in traditional Chinese medicine for thousands of years. It's a diaphoretic herb that decreases fatigue and weakness and is potentially valuable for depression. It's also helpful for digestion, and acts as an anti-inflammatory.

- The Bach flower remedies wild rose, larch, mustard, gorse and gentian help alleviate feelings of apathy, resignation, despondency, inferiority, despair, hopelessness, discouragement, self-doubt and intense descending gloom.

- Sunlight is vital for both physical and emotional health. Try to get 15 minutes of sunlight on your uncovered eyelids daily (no glasses) in the early morning or late afternoon. In the absence of sun, try sitting next to a multi-tube fluorescent light box (at least 2,500 lux) for 30 minutes each day upon waking.

- Massage is often more effective than talk therapy for reaching and healing hidden traumas and relieving depression. Even a single session can have a dramatic effect.

- Stand tall, smile with your whole face and breathe deeply. You'll either start feeling happier or make your rage or grief more visible and more easily accessed.

- To energise when depressed you can sigh deeply many times; hold your arms out in front of you for several minutes; bounce up and down on the balls of your feet. Try it!

Foods that Fight Depression

Grapefruit: This is great for boosting liver function and easing depression. The more toxins your liver is exposed to, the more easily its detoxification systems are overloaded. If the liver is sluggish, excessive amounts of toxins find their way into the bloodstream. This can affect the function of the brain, causing unpleasant and erratic mood changes, a general feeling of depression, 'foggy brain' and an impaired ability to concentrate or remember things.

Artichoke: This is liver protective and also has a bile-producing, and bile-moving, effect on the liver. When bile lingers in the liver, it irritates the tissue, creating inflammation and decreasing the ability of the liver to carry out its function so you're more likely to feel tired and depressed.

Watermelon: Studies indicate that red-pigmented, lycopene-rich foods, such as watermelon, tomatoes and papaya, improve liver health. A healthy liver is essential for detoxification and physical, emotional and mental health and wellbeing.

Sunflower seeds: Minerals are essential for the growth and functioning of the brain. Selenium (high in sunflower seeds, seafood and seaweed) has been shown to improve mood significantly. Other sources of selenium include brazil nuts, tuna, and wholegrain cereals.

Foods that Fight Depression (Cont.)

Oily fish and flaxseeds/linseeds: Fatty acids regulate memory and mood. Sixty per cent of the brain is made of fatty acids. The omega 3 types (DHA and EPA) are essential to the optimum performance of your brain. These are found in oily fish – such as mackerel, tuna, herring, salmon and sardines – as well as other foods such as avocado, olives, raw nuts and seeds and their cold-pressed oils. All these foods contain good mood stimulants, and it's been discovered that levels of depression can be improved by introducing these healthy fats to your diet. Omega 3 fats are also excellent intelligence and memory boosters. If you don't eat fish, try some hemp or flaxseeds/linseeds instead.

Lentils: These are an excellent source of B vitamins and folate. Folate deficiency has been linked to an increased risk of depression, and deficiency in B vitamins increases the risk of anxiety, insomnia and mood swings. (Folic acid is manmade from folate.)

Water: The body deteriorates rapidly without water, and dehydration is a common cause of tiredness, poor concentration and reduced alertness. So ensure you get your recommended eight glasses a day!

Digestive problems

Oestrogen and progesterone affect the speed at which food moves through your intestines. Progesterone reduces movement so that bowel movements become dry, pebble-like and infrequent while oestrogen speeds them up. Digestive problems may therefore be another common menopause symptom. Eating while stressed, overeating or eating too many 'junk' foods all contribute to unhealthy digestion. Another common cause of poor digestion is simply eating too fast. The most effective natural remedy is a healthy, fibre-rich diet, but the following may also help:

- Make sure you drink plenty of water. Drinking hot water with lemon juice in the morning will encourage regular bowel movements and ease constipation.
- Peppermint and fennel teas after a meal can ease digestion

and reduce trapped wind. Ginger as tea or in capsule form aids digestion and helps prevent the formation of abdominal gas. It's also great for easing nausea. Brew a cup of ginger tea and drink daily.

- If you have diarrhoea, avoid alcohol, caffeine, milk and dairy products until it has subsided. Try some potassium-rich banana, apple sauce, rice and dry toast until you feel better to help restore balance to your body. You can also use live yoghurt to replace beneficial bacteria in your intestines. Don't take any anti-diarrhoea medications until you've given these recommendations a chance to work.

- Chew your food slowly and thoroughly to encourage proper digestion. Before you begin a meal, start with a few cleansing breaths and breathe fully as you eat. Try to avoid distractions when you eat, like the television.

- If you have intestinal cramping and gas all month long in spite of these remedies you may have irritable bowel syndrome, a disorder that requires medical attention.

- If you get nausea along with digestive distress try drinking chamomile tea three times a day. Vitamin B6 can also help quell nausea. Increase the amount in your diet or take a supplement.

- If stomach acid is a problem, a cup of liquorice root tea has been shown to be effective.

- Acupressure has been found to be effective in reducing nausea. You can purchase acupressure bands to be worn around your wrists in many chemists.

- Lactobacillus acidophilus relieves chronic constipation and may be used freely. Capsules, or plain unsweetened yoghurt containing live and active culture, will help relieve digestive and gas pain, as well as restore good levels of beneficial bacteria to the digestive tract.

- Psyllium seeds are a healthy way to keep the colon healthy and clean in cases of constipation. The seeds are covered with mucilage that swells into a gummy, gelatinous mass when it absorbs fluid in the intestines, thus lubricating the gut wall. The increased bulk stimulates the gut wall, encouraging peristalsis.

- Don't use bran as a remedy for constipation as it can prevent the absorption of calcium and other nutrients.

Disorientation and clumsiness

Studies suggest that fluctuating hormone levels can cause lack of coordination, poor concentration and clumsiness, so you may feel more accident-prone and forgetful. For example, you may need to read a page over and over again to get the sense of it, or you may find yourself daydreaming when you need to be concentrating. Bear in mind that menopause isn't always to blame. Difficulty concentrating and becoming absent-minded may also be related to poor diet, lack of exercise, fluid retention, lack of sleep and stress. The following natural therapies should help:

- Pay particular attention to eating little and often and cutting down on stimulants such as caffeine, nicotine and sugar to ensure that your nervous system isn't being overworked by too much adrenaline.
- Make sure your diet is sufficient in B vitamins, especially vitamin B5 found in foods such as whole grains, brown rice, wholemeal bread, legumes, broccoli and tomatoes. Vitamin B5 is essential for optimum functioning of your nervous system. If lack of coordination is a real problem you may want to supplement with an additional 50mg of vitamin B5 a day on top of your multivitamin and mineral.
- Make sure your diet is sufficient in iron as low iron levels are associated with memory problems and poor coordination.

- Regular exercise also helps to keep you alert and sharp and can improve your concentration too. A brisk walk in the fresh air every day for around 20 minutes will tone up both your mind and your body.
- Learn a relaxation technique to give your nervous system a chance to repair and relax. Just a few minutes a day of relaxation is enough.
- Try some essential oils to soothe your mind and body and reduce unhelpful stress. Melissa, lavender and chamomile all have a calming effect that can help problems that contribute to clumsiness.
- Research has shown that ginkgo biloba can improve concentration, memory and reaction time. Ginkgo helps deliver oxygen to your nerve cells and your brain. A study in *The Lancet* showed that ginkgo can improve blood flow to the head. If mental and/or physical disorientation is a problem, you may want to take a tincture of ginkgo for a period of three to four months. Remember that herbs take a few weeks of daily use to create an improvement.
- Practise yoga and meditation to help improve concentration and alertness. While you're in a relaxed state, try counting backwards from 100, silently and slowly, as this will help stimulate circuitry in the brain. As your concentration improves, start to count back from 200 or even 500.
- It's a case of use it or lose it with your brain. Contrary to popular belief, brain power doesn't decrease as you get older, and studies show you can be just as sharp in your 60s as your teens. The secret is to use your brain and keep it active. So if you do find yourself becoming forgetful, keep your brain alive with new interests and challenges. Try your hand at crosswords or a sudoku every day.

Fatigue

Tiredness or fatigue is one of the most common symptoms reported by women before and during menopause. All the natural therapies given in this book should help boost your energy levels but the following may be particularly helpful:

- Make sure you balance your carbohydrate load with some low-fat protein to avoid the sugar highs and lows that cause fatigue. In fact, balancing your blood sugar levels is the best way to fight fatigue and boost energy.
- Step up your exercise routine as women who exercise regularly tend to feel more energised than those who don't.
- Eat foods that are high in fatigue-fighting potassium and magnesium. Prime sources include fruits, green leafy vegetables, nuts, seeds and beans. You also need to make sure you're getting enough iron. Foods rich in iron include wheat germ, dried fruit, shellfish, sardines, red and dark-green fruits and vegetables. If you're a vegetarian you may want to take kelp supplements.
- The B vitamins are crucial if you feel tired as one of the symptoms of a deficiency in the major B vitamins is lack of energy.
- Co-enzyme Q10, a substance present in all human tissue, is a vital catalyst for energy production, and if you're deficient you may feel tired. Food sources of co-enzyme Q10 include fish, organ meats (like liver, heart or kidney) and the germ portion of whole grains. You may also want to take 30mg a day of co-enzyme Q10 over a period of three months.
- Ginger can boost energy levels. Use it fresh in your food as a quick pick-me-up. Cinnamon is another energy-boosting spice.

- Aromatherapy oils such as basil and rosemary can be helpful for mental and physical fatigue. Both are stimulating and renewing, and you may want to add a few drops to your bath or use in a vaporiser.
- Refer to the recommendations for stress-busting on page 74 and and getting a good night's sleep on page 182, as stress and lack of sleep can cause fatigue.
- If your fatigue persists you may want to rule out hypertension, diabetes, candida, thyroid problems, anaemia or a food allergy. Consult your doctor.

Fatigue-fighting Super Foods

Grapes: The energy-boosting value of grapes is due to their high magnesium content. Magnesium is essential for energy production; deficiency has been linked to fatigue and muscle weakness.

Hemp seeds: These are power-packed with essential fatty acids needed for energy production. They are needed to make prostaglandins, a hormone-like substance crucial for fat-burning and stamina.

Broccoli: The range of B complex vitamins and the energy-boosting nutrients magnesium and iron can be found in fresh green (preferably raw) vegetables, such as broccoli, asparagus and spinach. Deficiencies in B vitamins, magnesium and iron are associated with energy slumps. Broccoli is also a good source of co-enzyme Q10 (*see opposite*).

Sprouts: When seeds are sprouted their nutritional power swells. The result is an energy-boosting super food. They help improve, revitalise, strengthen, regenerate and enhance the human condition. Sprouts contain a high concentration of anti-ageing, fatigue-fighting antioxidants as well as all the trace minerals, plus protein, enzymes and fibre.

Yams: These are packed with energy-boosting nutrients: calcium for strong bones; magnesium and potassium for energy production; folic acid and the antioxidant immune-boosting vitamin C. Their complex carbohydrate and fibre content also has a steadying effect on blood sugar, ensuring that your energy supply is constant throughout the day.

Hair problems

Since hair follicles need oestrogen, bad hair days can become the norm during the menopause. Problems may include dullness, dryness, split ends, poor growth, thin patches, hair loss and dandruff. You might notice more hair in your brush or that your hair is becoming drier and more brittle. You might also notice a thinning or loss of pubic hair. A gradual loss or thinning of hair without any accompanying symptoms is common during menopause, and the tips below may offer relief. However, hair loss accompanied by general ill health requires your doctor's attention.

- Hair loss can be made worse by nutritional deficiencies, especially a lack of iron, vitamins B, C and E, zinc or lysine (an amino acid). Follow the diet recommendations in this book. Consider bumping up the amount of iron-rich foods you eat from lean organic meats, apricots, dark-green and dark-red vegetables.
- Make sure you don't go short of essential fats and water. Dry hair that lacks shine and breaks easily is often a sign of a lack of essential fats. Since hair is 98 per cent protein, make sure you're eating enough lean fish and poultry or vegetarian sources of protein.
- Egg yolk and green peas are rich in an important B vitamin called biotin. (Avoid foods containing raw eggs. Raw eggs don't only pose the risk of salmonella but are also high in avidin, a protein that prevents biotin being absorbed. Cooked eggs are fine.) Biotin is a major component in the natural hair manufacturing process. It's essential not only for growing new hair, but also plays a major role in the overall health of skin and nails. It appears to metabolise fatty acids, a valuable growth factor in numerous processes in the body including the hair. Biotin is also seen as an aid in preventing hair turning grey. Include in your diet foods rich in biotin and use hair-care products containing biotin. Good food sources

include brewer's yeast, brown rice, green peas, lentils, oats, soya beans, sunflower seeds and walnuts.

- Try to avoid sugar and sugary products lacking in nutrients.
- Scalp massage – easy when you're shampooing your hair – can be useful, especially when combined with essential oils. Scottish researchers found that 44 per cent of alopecia patients massaging their heads daily with a mix of thyme, lavender, tea tree and cedarwood oils in a carrier oil reported a big improvement in their symptoms over seven months compared with just 15 per cent of those using carrier oils alone.
- Some natural practitioners prescribe the mineral silicon to prevent hair loss. Horsetail is a good source of silicon.
- Treat your hair gently. Use a soft brush and don't blow dry or curl your hair. Apple cider vinegar and sage tea make a good rinse and help make hair shiny. Use only natural products on your hair. Check out your local health food store for natural shampoos and conditioners.
- Liquorice extract taken orally or used topically in a cream from a traditional Chinese medicine practitioner may help prevent hair loss.
- Nettle tea may improve the quality of your hair. For extra shine, try rinsing your hair with nettle tea that has been strained and cooled. For dark hair, adding a teaspoon of vinegar or rosemary can add shine. The calming herb chamomile is traditionally used to lighten and brighten blonde hair.
- For thinning hair, try eating more iodine-rich foods like seaweed and taking a sea kelp supplement.
- Regaine, available from your pharmacy, is for women with a family history of hair loss who have a general thinning of hair at the top of the scalp. If you are thinking of trying Regaine, be sure to consult with your doctor first as it's not recommended for women with high blood pressure. It may also interact with certain medications.

Excess Hair

If you're suffering from excess hair on your chin, upper lip, back or shoulders, this could simply be related to the drop in oestrogen levels at menopause. However, for some women it could indicate an excess of androgen or male hormone, and a condition called hirsutism that can manifest as a symptom of polycystic ovaries (PCOS). Studies show that with a healthy diet and weight loss, symptoms of PCOS – such as hirsutism – decrease. Exercise can also improve hirsutism because the fitter you become, the lower your body fat and the better your insulin and glucose control. This in turn reduces the amount of testosterone your ovaries produce.

Shaving is the easiest way to remove unwanted hair; try a double-edged razor for the closest shave. Contrary to popular opinion, shaving doesn't cause hair to grow back faster or coarser. If you're spending too much time plucking, waxing and shaving, you need to seek advice from your doctor for hormonal therapy in addition to your basic healthy diet.

Headaches

Some women find that menopause brings relief from a lifetime of migraines, and others find that migraines appear for the first time during menopause. Many women who get migraines stop having headaches when they fall pregnant so the link between headaches and hormonal change is clear. Migraines have often been found to be a side-effect of HRT. The following recommendations may help:

- Drink plenty of fluids as dehydration can trigger headaches.
- Missing meals or nutrients can trigger a headache whether you are approaching menopause or not so make sure you don't leave more than a few hours between meals and snacks.
- See if you can find a pattern or a trigger to your headaches. When you get a headache, note what you ate, when you ate and how you felt when you ate. Watch out especially for foods such as cheese, red wine, chocolate,

citrus juice or fruit: these contain tyramine, phenyle-thylamine and histamine which can all trigger headaches. Unfortunately, symptoms often don't hit you immediately after eating these foods, so you need to keep a diary for several weeks to notice a pattern. Typical tension headache triggers include stress, fatigue, too much sleep, lack of exercise and activities that require repetitive motion such as chewing gum or grinding teeth.

- Magnesium helps your muscles to relax and a deficiency can trigger headaches. Make sure your diet includes foods such as leafy green vegetables, nuts and seeds, bitter chocolate, soya beans and whole grains. One study showed that women who took 300mg of magnesium twice a day reported fewer headaches than those who did not.
- Make sure your diet is rich in essential fatty acids, especially omega 3. Another study suggested that migraine sufferers showed a significant reduction in symptoms when they took omega 3 fish oils every day.
- It's best to avoid over-the-counter painkillers as many contain caffeine and you can also develop intolerance to them.
- Learn to relax. Try to regard headaches or migraines as evidence that the body needs time to be alone, to recharge. By reducing muscle tension you may be able to ward off a fair number of headaches. Sit or lie down in a dark, quiet room for 20 minutes and sleep, if possible, until the headache is gone.
- Regular exercise and stretching can prevent many tension headaches.
- Treat yourself to a neck, shoulder and head massage. Whether it's a traditional massage or acupressure, releasing physical tension and improving circulation can promote feelings of wellbeing and even prevent headaches. Simply rubbing your temples can relieve pain.
- Putting an ice pack on the area where the pain is focused can ease the pain. In some cases a warm bath can make

headache sufferers feel better, especially if an essential oil such as lavender is added. Other helpful oils include rosemary, which can stimulate blood supply to the head, and eucalyptus and chamomile to ease pain. Add a few drops to your bath or make up a massage oil.

- Some women find that orgasm can help get rid of headache as it opens up the blood vessels, whereas others find that it can bring on a headache.
- Many women find that acupuncture or homeopathy are useful treatments for headaches and migraines.
- If you have a tension headache and can't get to a dark room to relax, put your hands around the back of your head and drop your chin onto your chest. Press your chin down and hold for a minute. Then use your hands to turn your head to the right and hold for a minute. Then turn back to the centre and hold for a minute, then to the left and then back to the centre, again for a minute.
- One study showed that 70 per cent of migraine sufferers had less frequent attacks when taking the herb feverfew. The herb milk thistle may also be beneficial as it improves liver function.
- Don't ignore headaches that recur frequently. They could be a sign of an underlying health problem. If you have tried various DIY measures to no avail or your headaches become more intense or persistent, ask your doctor for advice.

Heart palpitations

Heart rates of up to 200 beats per minute may accompany hot flushes during the menopausal years. These palpitations aren't necessarily indicative of heart disease. They may be triggered by electrolyte imbalances from fluid loss, or by strenuous exercise and strong emotions.

- Breathing slowly and deeply for two to five minutes often brings about a heartbeat that is even and quiet.

- When a heart palpitation comes on, particularly if it's a fast, regular rhythm, try lying on the floor and elevating your legs and feet. Keep your hips close to the wall, and rest your feet on the wall. This makes blood rush down to the heart, returning the rhythm to normal. Please talk to your doctor before attempting this remedy.

- Fish oils and omega 3 fatty acids have been studied for heart arrhythmia more than any other natural supplements. Fish oils stabilise cardiac cell membranes.

- Mineral-rich herbal infusions of fresh, organic grape juice – or just eating grapes – have been found effective for palpitations caused by hot flushes and night sweats.

- Valerian root tea may slow and ease a racing heart.

- Rose flower essence is said to calm and steady the heart.

- Bear in mind that after menopause heart disease becomes as common in women as in men. If you suffer from other symptoms such as dizziness, headaches or blurred vision, have your blood pressure checked as you could have hypertension, a precursor to heart problems (*see below*).

High blood pressure

High blood pressure – hypertension – is a risk factor for heart disease. Blood pressure is the pressure of blood in your arteries. The higher your blood pressure, the greater your risk of developing narrowed arteries which can lead to heart problems, kidney disease and strokes. The good news is that if your blood pressure is high, it can be lowered by making changes to your lifestyle – such as improving your diet, exercising and losing weight – and, when needed, with tablets.

In general, if your blood pressure is not dangerously high, your doctor will wait for up to six months before starting you on anti-hypertensive medication. This will give your body a chance to lower its blood pressure through lifestyle and dietary changes.

- Lose weight if you're overweight. Eat a low-fat, high-fibre diet rich in fruits and vegetables, according to the Menopause Diet guidelines. Be especially careful to monitor your salt intake and keep it below 4mg a day. Garlic and onions haven't been found conclusively to affect blood pressure, but they are tasty substitutes for salty seasonings.
- A diet low in magnesium may make your blood pressure rise but doctors don't recommend supplements. You can easily get the daily recommendation of 500mg from the foods you eat. Magnesium is found in wholewheat bread, wholegrain cereals, green leafy vegetables (like broccoli, chard, spinach, okra and plantain), nuts, seeds, tofu, soya milk, beans, dry peas and seafood (oysters, scallops, mackerel and sea bass – prepared without added fat).
- Potassium helps prevent and control high blood pressure. Foods containing potassium include lean pork, lean veal, fish (catfish, cod, flounder and trout – not fried or made with added fat), low-fat or skimmed milk, yoghurt, dried peas, dried beans, green beans, apricots, peaches, bananas, prunes and prune juice, orange juice, lima beans, stewed tomatoes, spinach, plantain, sweet potatoes, pumpkin, potatoes and winter squash. Plan your meals so you eat 4,700mg of potassium per day.
- Make sure you get enough essential fatty acids and calcium.
- Watch your caffeine intake.
- If you drink alcohol, do so in moderation.
- Exercise aerobically. Walk for 30–45 minutes at least three or four times a week. Thirty minutes every day is ideal.

- Give up smoking.
- Reduce your stress levels. Stress causes your arteries and veins to constrict.
- Buy an at-home blood pressure monitor and check your blood pressure frequently. Record the results in a notebook.
- Check your cholesterol level once a year and record it in a notebook. High blood cholesterol can narrow arteries and make you more prone to hypertension.
- If diet and lifestyle measures are not effective or your blood pressure is dangerously high your doctor will prescribe medication, usually a diuretic or an anti-hypertensive drug. Diuretics reduce your circulating blood volume, decreasing the workload on your heart and blood vessels. Anti-hypertensive drugs help dilate the blood vessels. If the medications cause you to gain more than two pounds, tell your doctor.
- Diuretics will cause you to urinate more frequently, which has a tendency to deplete your blood potassium. Eat foods high in natural potassium, such as bananas, dried apricots, tomatoes and potatoes boiled in their skins.

WARNING

As a woman grows older, her chance of having high blood pressure becomes greater than a man's. You may have had normal blood pressure most of your life, but after menopause your chance of getting high blood pressure increases considerably.

Although some women may experience headaches, dizziness, loss of libido or blurred vision, most often high blood pressure presents no symptoms and you may be completely unaware that you have hypertension until something happens that requires medical attention. Regular blood pressure checks should be a part of every woman's routine health screening.

Hot flushes

Hot flushes are among the most common and uncomfortable symptoms of menopause, but their frequency and severity can vary from woman to woman. They occur because the brain decides the body is overheated and does all it can to cool things down. Hormonal changes during and after menopause may also be involved.

During a hot flush, waves of heat sweep your body (and often the face), reddening your skin and promoting free perspiration. The reddening may be blotchy or even and the perspiration slight or copious. A hot flush may last from a few seconds to four or five minutes, occasionally 15 minutes, but rarely for more than an hour. The sweating may be so profuse that perspiration runs down your face, neck and back and there may also be heart palpitations. The following simple measures can decrease symptoms:

- Record your flushes so that you can avoid situations or foods that might trigger them. Situations and foods known to trigger hot flushes include:

  ♦ Spicy food (cayenne, ginger, pepper)
  ♦ Acidic foods (pickles, citrus fruits, tomatoes)
  ♦ Hot drinks
  ♦ Caffeine (coffee, black tea, cola, chocolate)
  ♦ Alcoholic drinks, including wine and beer
  ♦ White sugar
  ♦ Hydrogenated or saturated fats (meat, margarine)
  ♦ Stress
  ♦ Hot weather
  ♦ Hot tubs and saunas
  ♦ Tobacco or marijuana
  ♦ Intense exercise, especially lovemaking
  ♦ Anger, especially if you can't express it

- Don't wear synthetic fabrics and avoid clothes with high necks and long sleeves. Find ways to cool down such as keeping a flask of iced water near you or using a fan.

- Exercise directly decreases hot flushes by reducing the amount of circulating luteinizing hormone and follicle stimulating hormone, by nourishing the hypothalamus, and by raising feel-good endorphin levels (which plummet with hot flushing). As little as 20 minutes' exercise, five times a week, may reduce flushes significantly.

- Hot flushes deplete vitamins B and C, magnesium and potassium. Frequent use of red clover or oat straw infusions will help replace these nutrients. They can also be found in food or taken as supplements.

- Research has found that vitamin C and bioflavonoids strengthen capillaries and can ease hot flushes. Supplements that combine vitamin C with bioflavonoids can be found at most health food stores. Look for supplements that contain 500–1,000mg of vitamin C and 200–500mg of bioflavonoids per capsule.

- Essential oil of basil or thyme may ease hot flushes when inhaled, used in a bath or foot rub or mixed with massage oil. For a portable hot flush remedy, place a few drops of an essential oil or cologne on a tissue or cotton ball and wrap in cling film. Open and inhale for instant relief when a flush strikes.

- Dong quai has been found very helpful for menopausal problems such as hot flushes. It's also reported to help relieve mental and emotional upset.

- Chaste berry (Vitex) has been found to affect pituitary function and has many uses, particularly in regulating hot flushes and dizziness. Preliminary trials have also shown that femal, made from pollen extracts, has promise as a remedy.

- Some women find that acupuncture can help relieve hot flushes.

Insomnia

Sleeping problems are common during the menopausal years. They are caused by feelings of volcanic heat, arctic chills and powerful surges of emotion. Some women sleep restlessly, wake early, go for a walk and need a nap later. Others feel so tense when they lie down they can't seem to drift off, and wake achy and irritated.

Women who have normal levels of oestrogen fall asleep more easily than women who don't. They spend more time in the deep dream stage of sleep and wake more refreshed. Dreaming is important for feelings of rest and renewal. You can still sleep without oestrogen but you tend to wake up feeling less refreshed. Before rushing to your doctor for a pack of sleeping pills, try the following tried and tested self-help remedies:

- To increase your chances of a good night's sleep you need to program your body clock. Create a bedtime routine, going to bed at the same time every night. Read or listen to music, and then go to sleep. If you do find it hard to nod off, keep a journal by your bed as creativity can often surface in the midnight hours.
- Although big dinners will make you feel sleepy they also prolong digestion, which interferes with a good night's sleep. It's best to eat your biggest meal before mid-afternoon and have a light evening meal. Include some chicken, extra-lean meat or fish at dinner to help curb middle-of-the-night snack attacks.
- Dishes seasoned with garlic, chillies, cayenne or other hot spices can cause nagging heartburn or indigestion and lead to problems sleeping. Avoid spicy foods at dinner. Gas-forming foods and hurried eating also cause abdominal discomfort, which in turn interferes with sound sleep. Limit your intake of gas-forming foods to the morning hours, and thoroughly chew food to avoid gulping air.

- The amino acid tryptophan, found in soya, turkey and peanuts, helps the brain produce serotonin, a chemical that helps you relax. Try drinking some soya milk or eating a slice of wholemeal toast with peanut butter before bedtime.
- Avoid caffeine. Even small amounts of caffeine can affect your sleep. Try eliminating all caffeine-containing beverages. If you feel and sleep better after two weeks of being caffeine-free, then avoid caffeine permanently. You can try adding one or two cups after the two-week trial, but cut back if sleep problems reappear. A warm herbal tea, such as chamomile, can soothe and relax. It also makes you feel full, which might facilitate sleep.
- Alcohol might make you sleepy at first, but you'll sleep less soundly and wake up feeling exhausted. This is because alcohol suppresses a phase of sleeping called REM (rapid eye movement), during which most of your dreaming occurs. Less REM sleep is associated with more night waking and restless sleep. One glass of wine with dinner is about your limit, and try not to drink alcohol within three hours of bedtime.
- A glass of warm milk at bedtime can often help due to the action of calcium on the nervous system.
- Avoid vigorous exercise in the evening, although gentle stretching or a relaxing walk can improve your chances of a good night's sleep.
- Lavender is a well-known sleep remedy. Try using a lavender sleep pillow, or put a few drops of the essential oil on a cotton ball or handkerchief and tuck it into your pillow. You may find a lavender bath relaxing before bedtime. Add a handful of dried flowers or a few drops of essential oil with a carrier oil. You could also try rubbing a couple of drops between the palms, then cupping them over the nose for several minutes, breathing deeply.
- Oat straw has been found to relieve fatigue and weakness, particularly when there is an emotional component. By

soothing the nervous system, it can help make sleep more restful. It's considered a cooling and nourishing herb that eases night sweats, anxiety and headaches. One cup of infusion before bedtime, or sleeping on an oat-hull pillow, may lead to restorative sleep.

- Nettle tea nourishes the adrenals and may result in fewer sleep disruptions. Try using one cup or more four times a week.
- St John's wort is a gentle helper for sleep. Try one dropperful in a cup of fresh hops or lemon balm tea.
- Passionflower is an old remedy for nervous insomnia and hysteria, restlessness and headaches. Use 15–60 drops of the fresh-flowering plant tincture before bed to relieve ongoing sleeplessness.
- Valerian root has been used for centuries to induce sleep. Other herbs that have a sedative effect include catnip and chamomile.

Loss of libido

With the onset of menopause you may experience a loss of libido. Most menopausal women notice a change in the way their bodies respond to sex. Lack of lubrication can cause painful penetration; arousal is more subdued because blood flows less quickly to the genitals; and breasts are less sensitive to touch, again due to a decreased blood flow.

Although menopause can contribute to a loss of libido it's important to understand that it's far from being the only cause. Common factors include stress, fatigue, children, illness, too much alcohol, poor diet, and medical conditions such as hypothyroidism, which become more common in the menopausal years. Some of these contributory problems can be worked on to great effect, and a determined effort to put your love life higher on your list of priorities will help.

If you're not feeling as youthful, don't like the image in the mirror or you feel alone, menopause can be very frightening, but it need not be. As they enter the prime of their life, many women gain a new sense of self and feel sexier than ever before. The following tips should help kick-start your sex life:

- Eat healthily according to the Menopause Diet guidelines. Vitamins A and B, zinc and selenium are all crucial for libido. Exercise helps too, by boosting your mood and body image.
- Check your stress levels. In general, stress dampens libido. A stressed woman may blame a host of other factors for her symptoms without realising that stress is the real cause of the problem. Deal with commonplace stress by following the tips on page 74.
- Depression is another major inhibitor of sexual desire. Try to understand why you are feeling low so that you act appropriately when low feelings come. If you feel you can't cope alone, reach out for the support of family and friends or see your doctor for referral to a counsellor or therapist.
- Most sex therapists agree that sex begins in the head. In a way it's an idea that overtakes you, and your body's physical reaction follows. A key part of starting that sexual idea is setting the mood. Romantic music can help, as can low lighting, a candlelit bath or your favourite romantic or raunchy film. Devote more time to foreplay, exploring and discovering what you and your partner enjoy. If you haven't felt sexy for a while, touching yourself can also be a way to reconnect with your body as a sensual, sexual pleasure. Once you're back in touch with your own desires it can be easier and less daunting to connect with your partner's.
- Re-evaluate how you feel about your body. Remind yourself that your ability to become aroused, achieve sexual satisfaction and reciprocate is there no matter what

you weigh or look like. Stop focusing on what society tells you is beautiful and concentrate instead on what you find beautiful and pleasurable about yourself.

- Relationship troubles can also contribute to loss of sexual desire. If you don't feel listened to, respected or important, it's natural to respond with resentment, and that resentment can dampen libido. It's important to open the lines of communication with your partner so that anger can be expressed in places other than the bedroom. If the problem is severe, such as infidelity, you may want to go to a relationship counsellor.

- If you find the idea of sex unappealing or uncomfortable, talk to a sex therapist to discuss your health, upbringing, circumstances, any body image issues you may have and your relationship so that you can find ways to give yourself permission to satisfy your sexual needs. You might want to do this alone or you might find it's more productive to talk to a sex therapist with your partner.

- If you feel you haven't got time for romance, make time. Give it a higher priority in your life. However busy or stressful your life gets, try to make sure you have some 'couple time' when you can unwind together and talk about your day. Plan regular meals out, cinema trips or weekend breaks so that the two of you get some special time together away from the hustle and bustle of your daily life.

- The power of touch should never be underestimated. Being hugged or petted is necessary for our physical and mental wellbeing. A massage is an excellent way to help you and your partner relax, and put you both in the mood for sex.

- The less often you have sex, the less likely you are to enjoy it or look forward to it, so make time for sex in your life. Regular sex keeps your sex organs healthy and releases tension. If you haven't got a partner, masturbation is a positive way to explore your body and release sexual tension.

- Numerous herbal treatments are thought to help put sexual desire and drive back into your life. These include agnus castus, celery, wild oats, parsley and damiana.
- Practising kegel exercises (*see* '*Vagina and Bladder Problems*', *page 204*) can give you better toned pelvic muscles to grip your partner's penis and increase your enjoyment.
- If a dry vagina is causing problems in your sex life, refer to the section on page 204 on 'Vagina and Bladder Problems'.

Libido-boosting Super Foods

Almonds (and nuts in general) and oily fish: These are prime sources of essential fatty acids which help maintain a healthy balance of sex hormones in men and women. Nuts are also rich in the mineral manganese which is vital for ovulation and the maintenance of healthy testes. A lack of it leads to loss of libido.

Asparagus: Containing calcium, phosphorous, potassium and vitamin E, this definitely does a body good. It boosts energy, aids the urinary tract and kidneys and helps with sex hormone production.

Avocado: The Aztecs called the avocado tree *ahuacatl* or 'testicle tree'. Avocados contain high levels of folic acid, which helps metabolise proteins, thus giving you more energy. They also contain vitamin B6 and potassium, two elements that help enhance both male and female libido.

Bananas: This fruit contains an alkaloid compound called bufotenine which acts on the brain to improve your mood, self-confidence and possibly your sex drive. Bananas are also rich in vitamin B6 which is important in the manufacture of sex hormones.

Berries, such as strawberries, blueberries and blackberries: Not only are they rich in the sex hormone zinc, but they're also incredibly high in antioxidants which help optimise blood flow to the sex organs. Berries have the lowest glycaemic load of any fruit, meaning they provide sustained energy levels at only a few calories.

Libido-boosting Super Foods (Cont.)

Celery: This contains androstenone, a biochemical cousin of the male hormone testosterone and believed to be the principal chemical of attraction, or pheromone. The Romans dedicated celery to Pluto, their god of sex and the underworld, and crushed celery seeds (easily added to salads or breads) are said to be particularly potent.

Chillies: They may heat up your sex life too, due to capsaicin – the substance that gives a kick to peppers, curries and other spicy foods. Capsaicin stimulates nerve endings to release chemicals, raising the heart rate and possibly triggering the release of endorphins, giving you the pleasurable feeling of a natural high.

Cinnamon: This spice is thought to tone the kidneys and produce a strong flow of energy. Chinese medicine links it to virile sexuality. Studies have also shown that the smell of cinnamon can boost concentration and alertness, important for satisfying sex.

Cocoa: The emperor Montezuma used to drink chocolate before entering his harem, which gave rise to the belief that chocolate is an aphrodisiac. Dark chocolate (70 per cent cocoa solids) actually contains the stimulants caffeine and theobromine, plus phenylethylamine, which is a mood-elevator. Some researchers say that the chemicals in chocolate stimulate the production of endorphins – feel-good chemicals found in high levels in new lovers.

Figs and dates: These are high in amino acids, which are believed to increase libido. The shape of a fresh fig and the sweet, juicy taste are two tangible aspects that are highly pleasurable.

Garlic: Yes, you might need to stock up on some extra breath mints, but it'll be worth it. Garlic contains allicin, an ingredient that increases blood flow to the sexual organs. As such, it's a highly effective herb for increasing libido. If the odour just won't work for you, or you can't stand garlic, you can always take garlic capsules instead.

Ginger: One of the oldest medicinal spices in the world, it allegedly increases the blood flow to the genitals and therefore acts as an aphrodisiac. Try it in a spicy dish served with saffron rice. It can also be used as part of an aromatherapy blend for massage or a room scent.

Honey: This is an aphrodisiac due to its rich B vitamin and amino acid energy-boosting content. Bee pollen is made from millions of particles of a semen-like substance, and can help boost fertility.

Lentils: These are a good source of B vitamins, which are essential for hormone balance in women and healthy sperm count in men.

Libido-boosting Super Foods (Cont.)

Lychee berries: Not only are these a good source of libido-boosting vitamin B, they're also packed with vitamin C. Research has shown that vitamin C is good for healthy fertility in men and women.

Mango: The mango is known as the 'love fruit' and has been used as an ancient Viagra. The *Kama Sutra* recommends drinking the tropical juices before sexual play, and who can argue with the bible of love! This wonder fruit contains zinc, a natural sex aid, and sugar and nutrients for stamina. In India, mangoes are very important for couples and feature at weddings and other celebrations as a symbol of love and the joy of life.

Oats: These are a good source of the antioxidants selenium and vitamin E. Deficiency in these nutrients has been linked to infertility in men and women.

Oysters: These have several qualities useful for lovers. They are low in fat but high in protein, complex sugars and zinc. Zinc is a very important part of testosterone, the hormone that governs sex drive in both genders.

Pomegranates: Also known as the 'love apple', pomegranates are high in chemicals that can encourage arousal and lubrication.

Pumpkin seeds: These are rich in the mineral zinc, which is Viagra for men and women. Research has shown that zinc governs testosterone, which is needed for sperm production, and a woman's body prepares itself for sex more quickly if zinc levels are high.

Spinach: This is a source of iron. Iron deficiency is a common cause of infertility, low libido and fatigue in women. Spinach is also a good source of calcium, which muscles need to spasm and contract. Deficiency of this vital mineral will turn the fireworks into a damp squib.

Tuna and prawns: Known as the king of sexy foods, tuna can raise the libido and stamina. Prawns are rich in phenylalanine, a chemical that helps increase sexual appetite.

Lowering of voice

You may notice that your voice becomes deeper, sexier and richer as you approach menopause. This may be caused by an increase in male hormones or androgens circulating in your blood which have a masculinising effect on your body and voice. Another possible cause is hypothyroidism (an underactive thyroid), where the voice becomes deep, gruff and hoarse, accompanied by other symptoms such as hair loss, a tendency to feel cold and fatigue. If you are suffering from hypothyroidism, your voice will return to normal once medication begins. If you are concerned about the change in your voice, consult your doctor for a diagnosis.

Hypothyroidism

If you're feeling tired for no reason and suffer from headaches, low libido, mood swings, dry skin, hair loss, weight gain, high cholesterol, poor concentration and intolerance to cold, you may be suffering from hypothyroidism or reduced thyroid function. Basically, your thyroid gland isn't producing the right amount of hormones, and this is upsetting your body's delicate biochemical balance. Many of the symptoms of hypothyroidism mirror those of menopause so you may want to visit your doctor to rule out hypothyroidism.

If hypothyroidism is diagnosed, the aim of any course of treatment is to normalise thyroid function and restore good health. Standard treatment for an underactive thyroid involves daily use of the synthetic drug levothyroxine. This oral medication can restore adequate hormone levels and shift your body back into balance. Although most doctors recommend synthetic extracts, natural extracts – such as Westhroid and Armour hormone, containing thyroid glands from animals – are also available.

Other recommendations include a healthy, low-sugar diet as symptoms can be greatly alleviated through diet and weight loss. Avoid fluoride (including that found in toothpaste and tap water) and chlorine (also found in tap water). Chlorine and fluoride are chemically related and can block receptors in the thyroid gland, resulting in reduced thyroid function.

Supplements include:

■ Kelp, made from seaweed, because it contains iodine, the basic substance of thyroid hormones.
■ Vitamin B complex for thyroid function.
■ Brewer's yeast as it is rich in basic nutrients, especially B vitamins, as well as essential fatty acids, iron, vitamins A, C and E and the minerals selenium, manganese, copper, iron and zinc, which are all important for proper functioning of the thyroid gland.

A medical herbalist might include the herbs bayberry, black cohosh and golden seal in a tailor-made prescription to help with this thyroid condition.

Menstrual irregularities

The journey into menopause is typically accompanied by menstrual changes. Your cycle may become erratic, large clots may be passed during menstruation, or spotting may occur. You may begin to experience these symptoms in your late 30s or 40s.

- If the amount of blood is usual for you but the pattern is weird . . . that's menopause.
- If the cycle is usual for you but the amount of blood isn't . . . that's menopause.
- If you seemingly skip a period and then have a real drencher several weeks later . . . that's menopause.

Listen to your body. You'll become able to distinguish the normal 'abnormalities' of menopause from really unnatural bleeding that needs attention and treatment. Talk to other women. Keep records. You may find a certain regularity to your irregularity.

First and foremost, the Menopause Diet and Detox Boost will help balance your hormones and ease period problems. The following tips should also help:

- Progesterone-producing and hormone-balancing herbs to choose when menopausal periods come too frequently include chaste tree (Vitex) berries, sarsaparilla (roots), wild yam (roots) and yarrow (flowers and leaves).
- Oestrogen-producing and hormone-balancing herbs to choose when menstruation is scanty, early or irregular include alfalfa and red clover (flowers/leaves), hops (female flowers), liquorice (roots), sage (leaves), sweet briar (hips or leaf buds), pomegranate (seeds) and any herb containing flavonoids.
- Bear in mind that irregular or absent periods are also a symptom of a common hormonal imbalance in women

(affecting as many as one in ten) called polycystic ovary syndrome or PCOS. If you suspect PCOS, consult your doctor to discuss your options and treatment plan.

Polycystic Ovary Syndrome (PCOS)

Doctors don't know what causes PCOS, although many suspect the cause may be genetic. There may also be a problem with the way the body uses blood sugar (glucose). The hormones that control the ovaries and menstrual periods can become abnormal and tiny cysts may develop.

Women in their childbearing years can get PCOS. It often begins in the teenage years and doesn't go away, even at menopause. Usually, women with PCOS have irregular menstrual periods. After a while, some women stop having periods. Women with PCOS may also have trouble getting pregnant.

About 70 per cent of women with PCOS have extra hair growing in the sideburn area of their face and on their chin, upper lip, nipple area, chest, lower abdomen and thighs. They may get acne. About half are obese. Many women have a condition called insulin resistance where there are problems with blood sugar regulation, and this can make it hard for them to manage their weight. Some women with PCOS have no symptoms at all.

If you suspect you have PCOS, it's important that you visit your doctor as PCOS carries with it an increased risk of infertility, diabetes and heart disease. Blood tests that measure your hormone levels can help diagnose the condition. An ultrasound examination can show if you have cysts on your ovaries.

Weight loss, diet and lifestyle measures and herbal remedies, in particular agnus castus, have been shown in many studies to be extremely effective for women with PCOS. Medicine can also help with irregular periods, infertility, abnormal hair growth and acne. Consult your doctor.

- Heavy bleeding (flooding) is one irregularity that is typical among menopausal and perimenopausal women. Flooding is a response to changing hormonal levels, most notably progesterone. Excessive bleeding may, however, be linked to other medical conditions such as fibroids or ovarian cysts so it's wise to consult your doctor if a period lasts more than twice as long as ever before or if there is a persistent low back/pelvic pain.

- Foods rich in phytoestrogens can help ease heavy bleeding because they help keep oestrogen under control and prevent excessive build-up in the lining of the womb. Foods rich in vitamins A, B, C and zinc are also important for heavy bleeding but it's especially important to make sure you are getting enough iron. Ask your doctor to confirm whether or not you are anaemic. You might also consider including some iron-rich herbs in your diet. Try dandelion leaves, milk thistle seed, echinacea and peppermint. Eating them on the day you're bleeding heavily is best. Essential fatty acids can also control heavy bleeding.
- Avoid coffee as this increases menstrual flow, and don't drink black tea and fizzy drinks with meals as this reduces the amount of iron that is absorbed.
- Agnus castus is the single best herb for regulating the menstrual cycle. When taken regularly, it acts on the pituitary gland, releasing the hormones that regulate ovarian function. Lady's mantle is another herb often recommended for heavy bleeding or flooding.
- Chinese herbalists recommend cinnamon for keeping menstrual cycles regular and stemming heavy bleeding. If you are bleeding heavily, sip a cup of cinnamon infusion, chew a cinnamon stick or take 5–10 drops of tincture once or twice a day.
- Applying pressure to acupressure points for one minute of every 15 is thought to help ease problems like flooding. One point is located above the centre of the upper lip (under the nose), and the other is at the top of the head.
- Avoid aspirin, Midol and large doses of vitamins C or E as they thin the blood (as does coumarin) and may increase bleeding.
- Also avoid blood-thinning herbs such as red clover, alfalfa, cleavers, pennyroyal, willow bark and wintergreen.

Premenstrual Syndrome (PMS)

If you suffered from PMS in the past you're likely to experience more intense symptoms as menopause approaches, such as fatigue, anxiety, tearfulness, water retention, skin problems and insomnia. If you think your mood changes are related to PMS, you can confirm it by charting your symptoms for three months; if the mood changes occur in the two weeks before your period then it's PMS; but if they occur at other times in your cycle they're not PMS-related.

■ To ease PMS improve your diet according to the hormone-balancing guidelines in the Menopause Diet and Detox Boost.

■ Fluctuating blood sugar levels can make PMS worse so make sure you eat little and often and leave no more than three hours between meals and snacks. You also need to avoid refined carbohydrates in favour of wholegrain, wholemeal complex carbohydrates.

■ Many studies have shown the effectiveness of vitamin B6 for PMS. Women with PMS have also been shown to have lower than normal levels of magnesium and zinc, so you might want to consider supplementing for three months to see if this makes a difference.

■ The herb agnus castus has been widely studied in relation to PMS and shown to be extremely helpful in re-establishing a normal balance of hormones.

■ Exercise, preferably in the fresh air, is important for your general health and to eliminate PMS symptoms.

■ Watch your stress levels as stress makes PMS symptoms worse.

■ A commonly recommended natural therapy is evening primrose oil. Other natural therapies that may prove helpful include acupuncture, homeopathy and reflexology. Aromatherapists recommend the calming and balancing oils of ylang ylang, lavender and lemon grass, which you can drop into a warm bath.

Mood swings

Mood swings are a classic sign of low blood sugar. If you're prone to this symptom, the best advice is to eat healthy and nutritious meals and snacks throughout the day. Don't go for long periods without food, and avoid caffeine and foods packed with sugar. Other helpful recommendations include:

- Consider taking supplements of B vitamins, magnesium and omega 3 fish oil in addition to your multivitamin and mineral. B vitamins can help your body produce serotonin, the feel-good hormone. Magnesium is well known as nature's tranquilliser, and essential fatty acids are important for hormonal balance. Boosting your calcium intake may also ease irritability.

- Try some Siberian ginseng to boost your adrenal glands and help you deal with stress. Chamomile tea is also great for anxiety-related disorders.

- Try aromatherapy oils in a massage or a bath, such as relaxing lavender, mood-enhancing chamomile and rose oil or calming sandalwood and clary sage.

- If you're prone to angry outbursts, remind yourself that you do have some control over yourself despite the way you are feeling. Question your motives. When you feel angry, stop and ask yourself why you feel this way and if your anger is appropriate to the situation. If you can do something positive, do it; but if you can't do anything, release your stress by using the stress-busting techniques in Chapter 4. See also the advice on anxiety and depression in this chapter.

Mouth ulcers and bad breath

You may find that as you get older you're more prone to gum problems, bleeding and bad breath. You may also get mouth ulcers. Although they may seem small, mouth ulcers and sores can be extremely painful and make it difficult for you to eat, smile and laugh. They can also make you feel run-down and tired. Nutritional deficiencies in iron, vitamin B12 and folic acid have been linked to painful mouth ulcers. Vitamin C and zinc are also important because they can enhance immune function and aid wound healing. Other helpful strategies include:

- Stress is perhaps the most common trigger for mouth sores so pay attention to your stress levels.
- You can buy gel-like ointment from your chemist – like Bonjela – to apply directly to the ulcer. It sticks to the sore and provides relief. If your sore or ulcer doesn't heal, consult your doctor.
- If your ulcer is allergy related, consult your doctor.

How to find out if you've got bad breath

Halitosis – bad breath – is very common but it's not always easy to discover that you suffer from it. It's almost impossible to test yourself, and only your nearest and dearest might be bold enough to tell you. One good strategy is to persuade a trusted friend or relative to sniff your mouth on a number of occasions and ask them to be honest about what they find. Or you could always ask your dentist for a professional opinion. The following strategies are useful for dealing with bad breath:

- Maintaining good oral health is essential to reducing bad breath. If you don't brush and floss daily, particles of food remain in the mouth, collecting bacteria which can cause bad breath. Food that collects between the teeth, on the tongue and around the gums can rot, leaving an unpleasant odour so schedule regular dental visits for a professional clean and checkup.
- What you eat affects the air you exhale. Certain foods, such as garlic and onions, contribute to objectionable breath odour. Once the food is absorbed into the bloodstream, it's transferred to the lungs, where it is expelled. Brushing, flossing and mouthwash will only mask the odour temporarily. Odours continue until the body eliminates the food.

- Other causes of bad breath include smoking, gum disease and a dry mouth. Xerostomia – dryness in the mouth – occurs during sleep or if you've been speaking for a long time. The saliva is a special kind of mouth moisture that kills oral bacteria. Drinking water can help prevent a dry mouth.

- Bad breath may be a sign of a medical disorder, such as a local infection in the respiratory tract, chronic sinusitis, postnasal drip, chronic bronchitis, diabetes, gastrointestinal disturbance or a liver or kidney ailment. If your dentist determines that your mouth is healthy, you may be referred to your family doctor or a specialist to find out the cause of bad breath.

- Avoid sugar, citrus fruits and refined, processed foods. Also avoid chewing gum, lozenges, sharp sweets, mouthwashes, tobacco, coffee and any other food that may trigger mouth sores and bad breath.

- If you think you have constant bad breath, keep a log of the foods you eat and make a list of medications you take. Some medications may play a role in creating mouth odours. Let your dentist know if you've had any surgery or illness since your last appointment.

- Dieters may develop unpleasant breath from infrequent eating. Eating regularly is important as it stimulates the production of saliva, helping to keep the mouth clean.

Keeping your breath fresh

Mouthwashes are generally cosmetic and don't have a long-lasting effect on bad breath because they don't treat the cause. If you constantly use a breath-freshener to hide unpleasant mouth odour, see your dentist. If you need extra help in controlling plaque, your dentist may recommend a special antimicrobial mouth rinse. A fluoride mouth rinse, used along with brushing and flossing, can help prevent tooth decay.

You can banish bad breath naturally by using home remedies. Here are some useful herbs and tips:

- Wash your mouth with water, sage leaves, mint leaves and parsley to rid yourself of common bad breath.
- Frankincense, also known as *Boswellia carterii*, is a herb with antibacterial properties, mainly used to treat sores and toothache. Other natural breath-fresheners are cardamom seeds and tea made from fenugreek seeds.
- Try chewing parsley, cloves, fennel or anise seeds after meals.
- You can also chew some minty fresh-breath herbs like wintergreen, spearmint or peppermint. They are also soothing to the throat.

Night sweats

A hot flush at night is called a night sweat, and may be accompanied by feelings of anxiety or terror. You might wake up feeling hot and drenched in sweat. Not everyone experiences hot flushes, and only some of those who do also suffer from night sweats. Night sweats can occasionally be a symptom of stress or a disease not related to menopause so you should consult your doctor.

- Sleeping problems in menopause are often linked to night sweats. You may wake up so wet that you have to get up and change the bed sheets. A solution may be to keep a glass of water and a towel by your bed so you can cool yourself down with tepid water. A battery-operated fan and scented lavender water can also ease discomfort.
- Agnus castus is a great herb for many menopausal symptoms including night sweats and hot flushes since it acts to normalise your hormones.

- Skullcap is a good sedative herb; valerian and chamomile have soothing properties; and lemon balm can ease anxiety.

- Pantothenic acid, a B vitamin, boosts the functions of the adrenal glands which take over most of the oestrogen production when your reproductive system stops. If night sweats are causing insomnia, try taking 500mg a day until you get relief.

- Garden sage acts quickly, and a single cup of infusion may help stave off the sweats for a day or two. To make a sage infusion, put four heaped tablespoons of sage in a mug of hot water. Cover tightly and let it infuse for at least four hours. Strain and drink hot or cold. If you prefer you can look for sage tea bags at your health food store.

- Avoiding the same foods and situations that can trigger hot flushes can help alleviate the intensity and frequency of night sweats (*see page 180*). Also, try not to eat meals late in the evening.

- Relaxation is especially helpful because it can help calm your mind and body, normalising your metabolism and making you sweat less. Meditation and yoga have a similar calming effect.

Skin, nails and eyes

The lower levels of oestrogen at menopause can cause changes in your skin, nails and eyes. These changes may be due to the weakening of collagen fibres and the protein elastin which gives connective tissues their strength and flexibility. One of the most distressing changes is the appearance of wrinkles on the face. The weakening of nerve endings in the skin can lead to a condition called formication, an itchiness or intense tingling that feels as if insects are crawling across your skin.

Other changes that might be caused by collagen deficiency include:

- **Skin:** Dryness or oiliness, flaking, bruising easily, wounds healing slowly, patches of brown pigmentation and prominent veins
- **Nails:** Brittle nails, white spots on nails
- **Eyes:** Dark circles under eyes, red blood vessels around the corners of the eyes, small yellow lumps of fat on the white part of the eyes
- **Hair:** Dullness, dryness, oiliness, split ends, hair loss, dandruff
- **Gums:** Bleeding and soreness, bad breath
- **Mouth:** Cracks on corners of mouth

The following simple tips can help protect your skin, nails and eyes:

- Make sure you eat foods rich in vitamins A, B, C and E as well as zinc, magnesium, iron and calcium. (*See pages 225–229 for examples of foods rich in these nutrients.*)
- Drink plenty of water to keep your bladder, skin and hair healthy.
- Sulphur-rich foods such as eggs and onions and live yoghurt with bifidus and acidophilus bacteria help to rebalance the bacteria in your gut and can protect against skin inflammation.
- Regular exercise, especially outside in the fresh air, is helpful because it encourages hormonal balance and healthy blood flow to your face to help flush out toxins.
- Keep make-up to a minimum and cleanse thoroughly with a mild but not astringent skincare product. Harsh cleansers or toners with alcohol strip the skin of natural oils, encouraging it to produce more in response and increasing the chance of spots. Avoid soaps. Never leave make-up on at night and choose oil-free moisturisers and products – look for the word 'non-comedogenic' on

labels. Opt for loose rather than pressed powders, and powder blushers instead of creams.

- It's important to exfoliate at least twice a week, unless you suffer from acne. This aids skin renewal and improves its elasticity, which is what makes our skin appear young.
- If you get a tingling sensation on your face, first check that you don't have an allergic reaction to a food or to substances that come into contact with your skin, such as washing powder. Then consider these remedies to reduce your discomfort:

  ♦ Try using a cortisone cream or a calamine-type lotion.
  ♦ Cool compresses or a face cloth soaked in milk and water can help.
  ♦ Itchy skin is known to get worse with stress so why not try a relaxing massage?
  ♦ Apply cooled chamomile tea to the skin with a soft cloth.
  ♦ Avoid scratching, and use breathing and relaxation strategies when the urge strikes.
  ♦ Keep your fingernails short, smooth and clean.

- Evening primrose oil may be able to relieve the itchiness associated with dry skin. Some herbal specialists prescribe oral lavender for dry skin conditions.
- Protect your skin against the sun. Wear sun block when you go out in sunny weather. If you can, limit your sun exposure to the early and later parts of the day.
- Take special care of your nails. Have a manicure and a pedicure every couple of months.
- White spots on your nails could indicate a zinc or protein deficiency so increase your intake of foods rich in zinc and protein such as nuts, seeds and oily fish.
- If you have dark circles under the eyes, eat a healthy diet and get enough exercise and sleep. It's not entirely clear

why inadequate sleep results in dark circles but we've all seen it happen. For one thing, lack of sleep tends to cause the skin to become paler (thus increasing the appearance of darkness under the eyes), and reduces circulation. It's also believed that too little time lying down is a cause in itself. Determine how much sleep you need (it's usually seven to nine hours per night) and try to get that amount regularly for a couple of weeks to see if that helps. Remember that alcohol and drugs can adversely affect the quality of your sleep.

- Wash your face with cool to somewhat cold water in the morning or when puffiness occurs. The cold water will cause blood vessels to constrict, and thus reduce swelling.

- Apply cool tea bags or cucumber slices to your eyes daily. The tannin in tea bags has been shown to reduce swelling and discolouration, and cucumber slices have long been used to reduce puffiness and refresh the appearance of skin around the eyes. Lie down, preferably in the morning, and leave fresh cucumber slices or cool, damp, caffeinated tea bags over your eyes for about 10–15 minutes. (You can refrigerate tea bags overnight so they'll be ready.) Keep your eyes closed.

- Apply an eye cream containing vitamin K and retinol. Dark circles may be caused by a deficiency of vitamin K. Recent research has shown that skin creams containing these two ingredients reduce puffiness and discolouration significantly in many patients. Long-term daily use seems to have the greatest effect.

- Avoid rubbing your eyes. Red eyes and eye irritation are usually brought on by allergies, but not always. The rubbing irritates the skin and can break tiny capillaries beneath the skin, causing both puffiness and discolouration.

Anti-wrinkle Super Foods

When it comes to nourishing your skin, the best way to do it is from the inside.

Almonds: These contain essential fatty acids, which help keep your skin smooth and hydrated. They're perfect for warding off crêpy necks and flaky skin.

Avocados: Containing myriad nutrients and vitamins, avocados help to moisturise, exfoliate and enrich the skin. They're particularly rich in vitamin E, an essential anti-ageing antioxidant which helps protect the skin from free radical damage. Vitamin E is also considered by professional beauty therapists to be an essential ingredient in treatments that help reduce the appearance of ageing.

Broccoli: This contains sulphorophane, an active compound that may help repair sun-damaged skin by preventing harmful toxins reacting with skin cells. Broccoli is also a great source of vitamin A which keeps your eyes sparkling.

Cherries, blueberries, blackberries and grapes: All contain anthocyanin, an antioxidant that keeps the skin supplied with nutrients through blood vessels leading to the face, helping to prevent saggy jowls.

Kiwi fruit: The copper content of kiwis helps promote skin texture and colour and boosts collagen production.

Oats: These contain the trace element silicic acid, which is used to make the spongy cells that lie between collagen and elastin fibres. These cells make the skin full and plump, slowing down the formation of fine lines.

Oily fish: As well as containing omega 3 oils, oily fish is a great source of protein to regenerate collagen and elastin, essential for keeping the skin plump, supple and hydrated so you have a healthy glow. Good sources include salmon, mackerel, herrings and sardines. If you're a vegetarian, hemp seeds are also rich in protein and essential fatty acids.

Onions: The sulphur in onions is a powerful detoxifier that helps to clean your liver and get rid of toxins, leaving your skin clear and fresh looking.

Soya milk, lentils, bean sprouts and wholegrain cereals: These contain plant oestrogens, which help make lubricating oils and collagen in the skin for a healthier look. They also help repair collagen and elastin, which slow down the thinning of the skin and the formation of fine lines.

Sweet potatoes, tomatoes and spinach: Free radicals in the environment can speed up the skin's ageing and wrinkling process. Antioxidants in your diet can help counter free radical damage. The antioxidant betacarotene is present in sweet potatoes, lycopene is found in tomatoes and lutein is present in spinach. They all go into the skin and help reflect harmful ultraviolet rays, acting as a permanent sunscreen to keep your skin elastic and lubricated.

Vagina and bladder problems

Bladder and vagina problems are common during menopause. The bladder and vagina are close together and can both become thin and dry when there isn't enough oestrogen to keep them lubricated.

Bladder problems include discomfort in passing urine and frequent urination, even when there isn't much urine in the bladder. There may also be some dribbling because the sphincter muscle guarding the exit from the bladder becomes weaker due to low oestrogen levels. You may find that urine sometimes escapes when you laugh, cough or carry something heavy.

During and after menopause the walls of the vagina can become thinner and less elastic. Your vagina may become dry and sometimes itchy. It may take longer to become lubricated, which can make sexual intercourse painful.

Women who maintain a healthy weight and eat a nutritious diet generally experience few problems with vagina or bladder weakness in the menopausal years. There are also some natural therapies that may help vagina and bladder health:

- Make sure you follow the guidelines in the Menopause Diet and Detox Boost. Drink plenty of water to keep your bladder flushed out. Try cranberry juice too, especially if you are prone to cystitis. Exercise can help keep your vagina supple and lubricated, as can regular sex and masturbation. The saying 'use it or lose it' doesn't apply just to your brain; it apples to sex too. Some women still lubricate rapidly when aroused, probably because they continue to have sex once or twice a week.

- Kegel exercises can help strengthen your pelvic muscles, combat incontinence and make sex more enjoyable. To find out which muscles you need to use, stop urinating in midstream by contracting your muscles; these are your pelvic floor muscles. Use these muscles to perform a kegel: contract them and hold for a count of five and then relax. Repeat this 10 times at least five times a day.

- Before sex, put some sterile water-soluble jelly on your vaginal entrance and a small amount inside your vagina. Avoid douches, talcum powder, hot baths, perfumed toilet papers and bath oils and foams as they can irritate the vagina. Don't wash the inside of your labia with soap as it will dry out the skin. Spend longer on foreplay as it will help you to lubricate.

- Motherwort tincture (25 drops) or 1–3 tablespoons daily of safflower oil or flaxseed/linseed oil taken orally may increase vaginal lubrication and vaginal wall thickness within a month of use. Wild yam ointment may be the herbal equivalent of oestrogen cream in its ability to restore moistness and elasticity to post-menopausal vaginal tissues. Vitamin E in daily oral doses of 100–600 IU for four to six weeks has been found to increase vaginal lubrication.

- Acidophilus capsules inserted vaginally help prevent yeast infections and create copious amounts of lubrication. Insert one or two capsules about four to six hours before lovemaking. Eating plain yoghurt with active culture four to five times a week helps maintain healthy intestinal flora and vaginal balance.

- If you are experiencing incontinence try to retrain your bladder (in addition to the kegel cure, *see above*). Begin by allowing yourself one trip to the loo every hour for a week. The following week extend the time between trips by half an hour. Continue this pattern until you are able to hold your urine for three hours at a time. This exercise teaches your bladder to hold more urine and become less spastic when full.

- Don't be tempted to drink less if you are prone to incontinence. Restricting your fluid intake won't prevent leaks. In fact it can aggravate incontinence by producing highly concentrated urine that irritates the bladder. Drink lots of water instead. You'll know when you are well hydrated if your urine appears clear to pale yellow. If it's dark yellow you aren't drinking enough. Herbs that may ease urinary symptoms include uva-ursi, buchu, ginseng and dong quai.

Weight gain
(See Chapter 6.)

Beating the Lady-killers

The hormonal changes that take place before, during and after menopause can increase your risk of three lady-killers: osteoporosis, breast cancer and heart disease. (*See also Chapter 2.*)

Outwit osteoporosis

Also known as brittle bone disease, osteoporosis is a greater cause of immobility than strokes or heart attacks. Bones become weak and fracture easily, resulting in disability, pain, loss of independence and even death. Osteoporosis is caused by too little calcium in your diet and poor calcium absorption. The risk increases with age, especially after menopause. Other risk factors are a slight build, family history of the disease, early menopause and chronic bowel problems like irritable bowel syndrome and diverticulitis.

Although some of these risks can't be changed, there are many others you can change and plenty of ways you can defend yourself against the onset of this disease. It's never too late to start because diet and lifestyle changes can slow and reverse the symptoms at any age. In addition to the Menopause Diet and Detox Boost guidelines, the following recommendations can help reduce your risk of osteoporosis:

Change your lifestyle

Women who sit for more than nine hours a day are twice as likely to have hip fractures as those who sit for fewer than six hours. If you have a sedentary job or lifestyle you should build more exercise into your life. Activity is crucial because it helps build strong bones and muscles, so make sure you follow the Menopause Diet exercise guidelines (*see Chapter 6*). Don't become a gym junkie, though. Excessive exercising as well as dieting and overeating can increase the likelihood of developing osteoporosis.

Avoid faddy diets

Without enough vitamin D and calcium your body cannot defend itself against osteoporosis. Cutting out dairy produce – a good source of calcium – because of imaginary food intolerances or fear of fat is a factor in an increasing number of cases. Obsessive dieting is another bad idea as it deprives your body of the nutrients it needs to keep your bones healthy. While it's important to lose excess weight, your body needs some fat to produce oestrogen. Thin women, especially those who diet and over-exercise, are more likely to suffer from osteoporosis and/or other menopause symptoms.

Stop smoking and drink in moderation

Women smokers generally have lower bone density and, after the age of 40, they lose bone faster than non-smokers. Excessive alcohol consumption interferes with the way your body handles calcium, increasing the amount you get rid of and decreasing the amount you absorb.

Eat for strong bones

Calcium is a vital mineral for the formation and continuing strength of your bones and teeth. A diet rich in calcium is your first step in protecting yourself against osteoporosis. Low-fat dairy products are good sources; a glass of milk provides the 1,000mg of calcium you need daily. It's also present in broccoli but you need to eat 2.5kg to get the recommended amount while just 100g of low-fat cheese does the trick.

A sufficient calcium intake is only half the story as you also need to absorb it. To do that successfully you should avoid foods that can leach calcium from your bones. These include fizzy drinks and foods too high in salt and additives. Tofu, soya milk and beans contain silicon and natural plant hormones that are protectors of bone health as women approach menopause.

In addition to calcium you also need plenty of vitamin D as without it your body can't put calcium into your bones. Your body manufactures its own vitamin D when your skin is exposed to ultraviolet light from the sun, and 10–15 minutes' daily exposure without sun block is perfectly safe in the early morning or late afternoon. The best dietary source is oily fish, although there are small amounts in eggs and cheese. If you don't go out in the sunlight regularly you should take vitamin D supplements.

A strong skeleton also needs omega 3 fatty acids from flaxseeds/linseeds and fish oil, and vitamin K from green vegetables which is vital for hardening calcium in your bones. Magnesium, found in nuts, seeds and peanut butter, is another vital mineral because it helps your body absorb calcium and vitamin D. If you don't think you're getting enough calcium in your diet, take supplements and ask your doctor to assess your risk and determine if HRT is required.

Watch your stress levels

When you are anxious your adrenal glands pump out a number of hormones including cortisol, which can increase the risk of fractures. (*See the stress management tips on page 74.*)

Combat breast cancer

This is the most common type of cancer in women and the leading cause of death in women aged between 35 and 50. Your breasts are dependent on hormonal stimulation for their development, and while we don't know all the risk factors we do know that the hormonal fluctuations at menopause increase the risk. Other risk factors are a family history of breast cancer and having no children or having your first child in your mid-30s or later. Researchers believe that the months without a period during pregnancy and breastfeeding may reduce a woman's risk of breast cancer. This supports the data that suggests that early menopause lowers the risk factor as well. Consider breastfeeding instead of formula feeding.

Fortunately, the lifestyle and diet changes that can case symptoms of menopause exactly match those recommended for the prevention of breast cancer. Once again, menopause acts as an early-warning system, giving us both reason and motivation to self-examine regularly, to consult our doctors about regular screening and to make positive diet and lifestyle changes. Here are some suggestions for reducing your risk of the disease.

Pass on that last drink

Studies have determined that women who drink alcohol develop cancer at a higher rate. How much is too much? Based on studies, women who consume two to five drinks daily have about one and a half times the risk of women who don't consume alcohol.

Quitters do prosper – when it comes to smoking

Although a direct link between smoking and breast cancer hasn't been made, studies suggest that smoking at an early age can increase a woman's risk. Not only can it be a risk for breast cancer, smoking is a definite risk factor for lung cancer.

Watch your fat intake

Researchers believe a diet high in saturated fat increases the production of the kind of oestrogens that can trigger cancer. Reduce your intake of saturated fat (animal fat and hydrogenated vegetable oils) and try to keep to a low-fat diet. A diet low in fat not only decreases the risk of obesity, but it can also reduce your risk of breast cancer. We know that oestrogen plays a major role in the development of breast cancer. Fat tissue contains small amounts of oestrogen and may increase your risk. There have been conflicting studies about fat intake and breast cancer risk; however, all studies have concluded that obesity plays a big part in breast cancer development.

Get physical

Lack of physical exercise encourages obesity. Exercise decreases the type of oestrogens in the body that are related to cancer.

Check your breasts

Checking your breasts every month may not reduce your risk of developing breast cancer but it may help detect breast cancer early. The earlier breast cancer is found, the less aggressive the treatment needs to be. (*Refer to the breast self-examination tips on page 161.*)

Don't forget to have a mammogram – it's not a choice. Like the breast self-examination, a mammogram can detect cancer early. It's also likely to detect any lumps that cannot be felt.

Heal your heart

Heart disease is the number one killer of women in the UK and US. In fact, more women die from heart disease than all cancers combined, including breast cancer. While some risk factors are unavoidable, such as having a family or personal history of heart problems or oestrogen deficiency at menopause (oestrogen has a protective effect on the heart), there are plenty of steps you can take to lower your chances of getting heart disease.

Don't smoke

The American Heart Association names smoking as the most important preventable cause of premature death in the US. Smokers have twice the risk of heart attack as non-smokers, and are more likely to die from a heart attack. Fortunately, just two or three years after quitting, their risk of heart disease and stroke returns to normal.

Have your ccholesterol checked

Ask your doctor for a 'simple lipid panel' that shows your HDL (high-density lipoprotein), LDL (low-density lipoprotein) and triglyceride levels. If you have too many LDLs (also called 'bad' cholesterol), they begin to clog up your arteries. HDL, or 'good' cholesterol, can help carry cholesterol away from your arteries and out of your body but smoking, physical inactivity and obesity can lower your HDL level. Having a consistently high level of triglycerides (unhealthy fats) can signal an increased risk of heart disease. Your goal is a low LDL (under 130), high HDL (over 50) and low triglycerides (under 200). If your numbers are not in the healthy range, ask your doctor for advice.

Get your blood pressure checked regularly

Discuss with your doctor the best way to monitor your blood pressure: by visits to the surgery or using a home monitoring kit. High blood pressure makes your heart work harder, eventually leading to its enlarging and weakening. Additionally, the build-up of fat and cholesterol in the arteries accelerates, increasing your chances of developing a blood clot. High blood pressure usually produces no symptoms until the damage is done, so it's important to monitor yourself. Your blood pressure is considered high if it reads 140 over 90 or greater, and borderline if it reads 130–139 over 85–89.

Eat a healthy diet

Add foods to your diet that are low in cholesterol and saturated and trans fats because your body turns saturated fats into cholesterol. Consider nutritional supplements but check with your doctor if you're on medication. Some studies have shown that vitamin E may lower the risk of having a heart attack. Garlic and hibiscus contain antioxidants that may reduce cholesterol, and artichoke leaf and hawthorn reduce blood pressure. Try valerian and lemon balm for stress.

Ask your doctor about taking a low dose of aspirin each day. Aspirin helps prevent coronary heart disease, but taking it also has some risks.

Exercise regularly

Studies show that even moderate exercise, such as walking, reduces the risk of heart disease by improving circulation, enhancing efficient use of fats and sugars, and helping to lower blood pressure and cholesterol levels. Exercise at least three or four times a week on a regular basis for 30–40 minutes at a time.

Reduce stress

Your body responds to stress by making your blood pressure and heart rate higher. This means your heart has to work harder. Over time, high levels of stress can harm your health. If stress is a problem for you, try exercising more or use other relaxation techniques.

Lose weight if needed

Obesity exacerbates other risk factors, such as high blood pressure and high cholesterol.

Let a little love into your life

Simple things like laughing, holding hands or chatting to a friend can lower your blood pressure by 50 per cent say experts from North Carolina University.

Lighten up for Life

Now that you've read the Menopause Diet guidelines, you'll recognise where changes need to be made in your diet and lifestyle to maximise your chances of success. The challenge for you now is to get motivated, and then keep the motivation going so you stick with the plan long enough to see the benefits.

Finding the Motivation

You may think you want to lose weight but are you motivated enough to change? This motivation has to come from within. I'm assuming you're reading this book because you want to lose weight or manage your weight. Well, take that first step now by changing the way you think about food.

Stop thinking about food in terms of pleasure or pain and start looking at it as fuel. Food is fuel that can control your symptoms, prevent heart disease and osteoporosis, help you lose weight and maximise your chances of health and a long, happy life. Thinking about all the benefits you get from healthy eating is a powerful motivator. If you keep this in mind when you start to change your diet, your path will be much easier.

Below you will find some mindset-changing exercises that can be particularly helpful when you're starting a healthy-eating programme.

Glimpse the future

It's hard to change old habits but a good way to start is to conjure up powerful images of how you will look and feel if you *don't* make changes in your life. Perhaps you see a little old lady, bent almost double as she tries to cross the road? Perhaps you feel constantly low and tired? Perhaps the weight gain around your middle is so excessive that your partner can't put his arms around you any more?

This exercise also helps you focus on the real reasons why you are making changes in your diet. Thinking about weight loss and good health will make your future a happier place to imagine.

Think thin

Once you've started to get motivated it can help to see yourself slim, fit and healthy with shiny hair and soft skin. You can then link this vision of health and wellbeing with healthy eating and regular exercise. See yourself enjoying healthy foods. See yourself having the energy to exercise. You need to use this visualisation technique every day until it becomes a habitual way of thinking, until you start seeing yourself as fit, not fat, after 40. Spend time daydreaming, playing a movie in your mind in which you look and feel great. Watch that film over and over again whenever you need a boost.

Stay positive

You can also help yourself stay positive with daily motivational statements such as 'I'm feeling fit and healthy' or 'I'm looking and feeling good.' Affirmations like these won't make you slim but they'll give you that extra energy boost you need to keep going with the plan.

Reward yourself

When you do notice an improvement in your symptoms or in the way you look and feel, be sure to make a note of it. We often tend to dwell on the negative so give your body and mind a break and mull over the positive instead. Give yourself a pat on the back and remember that feeling by treating yourself to a new hairstyle, a night at the cinema, a relaxing bath, a visit to the countryside or a phone call to someone you love.

Sticking with the Plan

Once you've got motivated, remember to take your time with introducing changes to your diet and lifestyle. The dietary changes recommended in the plan are not a short-term fix. Rather, they're designed to get to the heart of the hormonal imbalances that increase the likelihood of weight gain and symptoms in the years approaching menopause. So start slowly and gradually. You are re-educating your eating habits for life, and small changes are the best way to lose weight and boost your health.

Although you'll see benefits within days or weeks of starting the plan, it will typically take around two months before you start to notice considerable improvements in your symptoms and weight loss. It can be difficult to stick to resolutions if you don't see immediate results but the advantage of taking things one day at a time is that you will see long-lasting results. Think of it like saving: if you look after the small things today (such as the daily decision to eat healthily and get some exercise) then the bigger things (such as weight loss and the reduced risk of heart disease and osteoporosis) will take care of themselves.

When you first start making changes it may well seem a bit time-consuming and uncomfortable. For example, if you're used to spending hours watching television, making the effort to exercise will be a shock to your system. Or if you rely on chocolate to get you through the day, replacing it with healthy snacks will be a wrench. It will take a couple of weeks before any change starts to feel comfortable, and experts reckon that most of us need 12 weeks to completely break old habits and replace them with new ones. But if you stick with it, you'll eventually find it difficult to imagine that you could ever have enjoyed such things. If you've ever given up sugar in tea or coffee you'll know that at first the drink tastes really bitter but soon (after around 21 tastings) you get to the stage where it would taste awful to you with sugar back in.

No matter how hard you try, there will be times when you slip back into old habits. Don't punish yourself when this happens. It's all part of the healthy-eating process. Just know in advance that setbacks will happen – they happen to everyone – and that they will pass. Women who try but fail are twice as likely to succeed next time. Just remember the 80/20 rule (*see Chapter 3*) and tell yourself that tomorrow is another day.

When it comes to the Menopause Diet, positive thinking and taking life one day at a time will get you a long way. A lot depends on your attitude. Thinking in terms of failure won't help so turn your thinking around. You *can* lose weight.

Seven Habits for Managing Your Weight at Menopause

1. Lose weight because you want to and not because you are trying to please someone else.
2. Find time to exercise, however busy you are.
3. Eat little and often: around five to six small meals and snacks a day with the biggest meal at lunchtime.
4. Drink plenty of water throughout the day.
5. Don't give up on your favourite foods, however unhealthy they may be. Eat them, just don't overeat them.
6. Aim for slow and steady weight loss by taking life one day at a time.
7. Regardless of what the number reads on the scales, find ways to feel good about yourself and your life.

Light Years Ahead

As menopause approaches you may not feel as optimistic as you once did about tomorrow and what the future might bring. At best, most of us feel ambivalent about getting older. In terms of your health and wellbeing, however, there really is so much to be positive about in the years approaching menopause and beyond.

Age 40–45: the best years so far!

Research tells us that when you hit the big 40 there's plenty to look forward to and celebrate. For starters, you can enjoy a guilt-free couple of glasses of wine a day. It could cut your risk of a heart attack by 60–80 per cent and even improve your brain power, according to research carried out at the Australian National University in Canberra. The study found that 40-year-old women who drank moderately (moderately is the key word here) had better verbal skills, memory and speed of thinking than those who didn't. This is because alcohol helps to eliminate harmful cholesterol from your arteries, improving blood flow to your heart and brain.

If you're short-sighted you might also find that your eyesight improves in your early 40s. As you get older your eyes suffer from presbyopia, which means you can't read small print close up and need to hold books and newspapers at arms' length. If you're short-sighted (objects a long way off are blurred) then presbyopia can balance it out. You won't have perfect vision but you may not need reading glasses, and your long-distance vision prescription won't be as strong as it was when you were in your 20s.

Best of all, 40 is the age when you blossom into your prime. Many women say that the early 40s are the best years of their lives, and that they wouldn't want to turn the clock back, even if they could. This is because many of us feel more confident and self-assured than ever before. There are many reasons for this but life experience has to be one of them. Also, with the difficult and intense baby and toddler years fading into the past, we're still enjoying our family and look young enough to earn decent salaries and get the most from life. And for those who delayed baby-making, the early 40s still come out on top as we've got the partying out of our system and can focus on what really matters to us.

Age 45–50: a great time to have sex and go blonde!
The later part of your 40s is all about adventure and experimentation, not just in the bedroom but in all areas of your life. With your confidence at an all-time high, life is more exciting and rewarding than ever.

You're most likely to be sexually adventurous at this age. Researchers aren't sure why, but it could be a powerful surge in hormones before menopause kicks in, or simply because your childbearing years are likely to be over and there's a heady freedom in having sex without the risk of pregnancy. You're also more likely to have overcome any body image problems and know what you like and don't like in the bedroom.

You also start needing less sleep. According to research carried out at Loughborough University's Sleep Research Centre, you need less sleep now than you did in your 20s and 30s. You start by needing about 30 minutes less sleep, and by the age of 70 you'll need up to three hours less sleep. This means you can stay up later at night without feeling the effects the next day, and you can use that extra time to have sex or do things you always wanted to do but haven't had the time or energy for before.

The late 40s are a great time to reinvent yourself with a new hairstyle and/or colour. Most 50-year-old women have around 50 per cent white hair. If you're one of them, don't fight it by dyeing your hair the colour it was when you were

30 – dark colours can look harsh. Go lighter, using the white hair as a guide to highlights. It's a great opportunity to find a look that really flatters your skin.

Age 50–55: all change

Most women experience the final stage of menopause at the age of 51. If you've always had heavy or painful periods, it really is a big plus. No more panty liners, tampons, painkillers, backache and worrying about contraception or PMS. So the onset of the change really is something to look forward to. Why not use the money you will save on some pampering? For example, you could have a bunch of mixed roses delivered to your door every month for five months or take to the shops and treat yourself to a pair of gorgeous, sexy shoes.

Your vocabulary range, use of language and problem-solving skills peak in your late 40s and early 50s, and life experience and general knowledge continue to contribute to your wisdom. Now is the time to write that novel, sign up for an evening class, learn a new skill or study for a degree or doctorate. Hang on to your brain power and exercise it by doing crosswords or puzzles and read a newspaper to keep up with current affairs.

If sex wasn't a priority in your life before it could be now. Contrary to the myth of sexual decline, some women – about one in six – report increased sexual desire after menopause, which may or may not be due to raised levels of male hormones.

Your energy levels are at an all-time high. If you are post-menopausal your ovaries have stopped producing oestrogen, the female hormone that causes mood swings and hot flushes. It's replaced with the male hormone testosterone, which can result in a surge of energy and be a real mood booster. You'll feel better than you have done for years. This energy high is a big boost that often gets lost in the hype about menopause moans. Why not use all that energy to train for a marathon or another physical challenge? There's no reason why you shouldn't be able to get your fitness levels back to those of a 35-year-old. Follow the Menopause Diet exercise guidelines (*see Chapter 6*). Training is brilliant for your health and you could shed 10 years in looks.

Finally, if you've always wanted perfect teeth, now's your chance. Braces aren't just for children. You can still straighten and whiten your teeth in your 50s and 60s and it can make a real difference to your appearance. Caring for your teeth is worth doing cosmetically and medically.

Age 55–60: slimmer and fitter than ever

Menopausal weight gain slows down around the age of 55 for most of us. As we've seen, you don't just have to accept putting on weight during the menopause. Although dieting won't work, healthy eating will and you can use the energy boost you get in the early 50s to take more exercise and rev up your metabolism. You could end up looking fitter and slimmer than you did 30 years ago.

Your improved energy levels will mean you are more active, and the more active you are the better your skin and muscle tone will be. You might also be able to bin the razor. Hair growth on your arms and legs slows down and becomes much finer – you'll find that you shave less and less. The downside is that hair might start to appear on your chin or upper lip but this can easily be dealt with by using laser treatment or electrolysis.

Your memory could be better than it ever was. Believe it or not, an overtaxed lifestyle could mean that you are more forgetful when you're younger than in later middle age. Research at the University of Michigan tested 121 people between the ages of 24 and 84 on how many remembered to take tablets when they needed to. The youngest fared worst because they were too busy and stressed. The older participants did better because they had more time and were more relaxed. So as you head towards 60 your brain could be sharper than ever.

And here's a fascinating thought: by the time you hit 60 you could find yourself living forever! Technology in our lifetime could well develop so that you go on and on. Clinical trials are already happening to repair molecular and cellular damage that ages mice. Who knows: in another 20 years that technology might be available for you!

Age 60 and beyond: the golden years

Life feels so much easier once you hit 60. Surveys have found that the most stressed-out group of people are commuters in their 30s and 40s. People over 60 have lower stress levels, regardless of whether or not they have retired. They also cited higher levels of contentment. Now, that's a big plus.

You could also experience your first orgasm in your 60s. Women over 60 are more relaxed about their sexuality; they have a sense of humour about their sex lives and aren't worried about looking or feeling silly. They have a now-or-never approach to sex, which is a real turn-on.

Last but by no means least, there's still time to change your body shape. In one trial, participants aged between 61 and 72 doubled their muscle strength over a 12-week period and had fitness levels similar to those of a 20-year-old. They reduced their waist size by two inches and their posture improved.

The Time of Your Life

There's so much to look forward to whatever age you are. Menopause is not an ending but a wonderful new beginning, and if you follow the Menopause Diet and lifestyle guidelines there's everything to gain and nothing to lose. So what are you waiting for? Get out there and have the fittest, healthiest, happiest and most exciting time of your life.

10 Golden Rules: Your Action Plan in a Nutshell

1. **Forget three meals a day:** Eat five to six small meals and snacks instead. Don't skip meals – especially breakfast.

2. **Get your five a day:** Make sure you have at least five daily servings of vegetables and fruit.

3. **Forget low-fat:** Ensure your diet contains sufficient essential fats, such as oily fish, nuts and seeds.

4. **Drink plenty of water:** Your body is around 70 per cent water so drink plenty (around six to eight glasses a day) to stay hydrated.

5. **Be nutrient rich:** Make sure your diet is rich in nutrients, and for an insurance policy take a multivitamin and mineral every day.

6. **Say the F-word:** Ensure you are getting enough fibre from good sources such as whole grains, vegetables and legumes.

7. **Stock up on soya:** Increase your intake of phytoestrogens, including soya.

8. **Reduce your intake of CASSSA:** CASSSA stands for caffeine, alcohol, salt, sugar, saturated fat and additives.

9. **Walk this way:** Exercise for 30 minutes once a day or 15 minutes twice a day. Get off the bus a few stops early. Take the stairs instead of the lift.

10. **Menopause, no sweat!** Have an upbeat, positive attitude to your diet and your life. Like fine wine you really can get better and better.

Essential Nutrients Guide

Vitamin A (Retinol)
Essential for healthy skin and eyes, it protects the body's cells against attack and builds up resistance to infection. Pregnant women should limit their intake.
Good food sources: Calf's/lamb's liver; carrots; cheese; egg yolks; fish; fish liver oils

Vitamin B1 (Thiamin)
Essential for the digestive and nervous systems, it helps us cope better with stress, stabilises the appetite and promotes growth and good muscle tone.
Good food sources: Hazelnuts; Marmite; oats; pork; wheat germ; wholemeal bread

Vitamin B2 (Riboflavin)
Promotes good health and is necessary for maintaining good vision, nails, skin and hair.
Good food sources: Calf's/lamb's liver; dark-green leafy vegetables; eggs

Vitamin B3 (Niacin)
Improves circulation and reduces high blood pressure and cholesterol levels. Helps maintain healthy skin, mouth and digestive system.

Good food sources: Chicken; dried beans and peas (cooked); fish; liver; Marmite; peanuts; potatoes; raisins

Vitamin B5 (Pantothenic acid)
Known as the 'anti-stress' vitamin as it improves the body's resistance to stress. It also helps make antibodies to fight invading germs and bacteria.

Good food sources: Beef steak; bran; broccoli; chicken; dairy products; eggs; milk; mushrooms; peanuts; pig's liver; sweet potatoes

Vitamin B9 (Folic Acid)
Works with vitamin B12 for the growth and reproduction of new cells. It is essential for the development of the foetus and helps prevent spina bifida. It can also help to regulate moods, sleep and the appetite.

Good food sources: Avocados; bananas; dark-green leafy vegetables; lentils; oranges; pig's liver; watercress; wholemeal bread

Vitamin B12 (Cobalamin)
Works with folic acid and is essential for the formation and regulation of red blood cells, preventing anaemia. It is necessary for metabolism and a healthy nervous system.

Good food sources: Cheese; eggs; fish; full-fat milk; shellfish

Vitamin C
Needed for fat metabolism, it also helps with iron absorption. It is essential to the health of the skin, hair, teeth, eyes, gums, bones and ligaments. It helps keep the immune system in order, protecting against colds.

Good food sources: Baked potatoes with skin; broccoli; cabbage; fresh fruit (especially citrus fruits); peppers; pumpkin; tomatoes

Vitamin D

Works with calcium to keep the blood and bones healthy and strong. It helps to maintain a stable nervous system and normal heart action.

Good food sources: Butter; egg yolks; liver; milk; oily fish

Vitamin E

Helps protect against age-related ailments, cancer and heart disease. It helps maintain a healthy circulation and normal levels of cholesterol and is needed for cell formation, especially in the skin.

Good food sources: Asparagus; cereals; dark-green leafy vegetables; nuts; soya beans; vegetable oils; whole grains

Betacarotene

Carotenoids, the best-known of which is betacarotene, decrease the risk of most cancers.

Good food sources: Apricots; avocado; broccoli; carrots; dark-green leafy vegetables; kale; peaches; spinach; spring greens; tomatoes; watercress

Boron

Despite being essential for normal growth and the hormone involved in bone metabolism, boron has yet to be added to the official essential nutrients list.

Good food sources: Almonds; asparagus; cabbage; figs; peaches; raisins; strawberries

Calcium

Creates and maintains healthy bones and teeth. It regulates the heartbeat and may be important in preventing and treating high blood pressure.

Good food sources: Baked beans; bread; dairy products (except butter); dark-green leafy vegetables; dried fruit; eggs; nuts; rhubarb

Copper

An essential nutrient for bone synthesis, it also makes sure that iron in the body is in the right form to be used in the manufacture of haemoglobin.

Good food sources: Beans; calf's liver; carrots; chocolate; lentils; nuts; olives; shellfish; wholemeal bread

Iron

Used to make haemoglobin, which transports oxygen from the lungs around the body.

Good food sources: Beans; beef; broccoli; calf's liver; dried fruit; fish; nuts; poultry; soya beans; spinach; whole grains; wholemeal bread

Lycopene

An antioxidant that helps prevent cell damage and repairs damaged cells, it may lower the risk of heart disease and some cancers.

Good food sources: Guava; pink grapefruit; tomatoes and tomato products (sauce, juice, ketchup); watermelon

Magnesium

Magnesium is needed for more than 300 biochemical reactions in the body. It helps maintain normal muscle and nerve function, keeps heart rhythm steady, supports a healthy immune system and keeps bones strong. Magnesium also helps regulate blood sugar levels, promotes normal blood pressure and is known to be involved in energy metabolism and protein synthesis.

Good food sources: Almonds; oatmeal; spinach; soya beans; halibut

Omega 3 Fatty Acids

These reduce the stickiness of the blood, making it less liable to clot and cause thrombosis. They also lower blood pressure and promote a healthy cardiovascular system.

Good food sources: Oily fish (like herring, tuna and mackerel); nuts; seeds

Omega 6 Fatty Acids

These regulate hormone production and stimulate skin and hair growth.

Good food sources: Oils from cereals; pulses; vegetables

Phytoestrogens

Although not officially an essential nutrient, phytoestrogens are included here because of their importance in easing menopause symptoms. These naturally occurring plant extracts exert an oestrogen-like influence on the body and can help ease hormonal fluctuations in women.

Good food sources: Brown rice; garlic; oats; legumes; parsley; soya

Selenium

An antioxidant, selenium boosts the immune system and combats the ageing process.

Good food sources: Cod; crab; dairy products; eggs; garlic; meat (especially liver and kidney); seeds; wholemeal bread

Zinc

An essential nutrient used by the body for the growth and repair of tissue.

Good food sources: Beef; canned fish; chicken; eggs; hard cheese; mushrooms; nuts; oysters; pulses; shellfish

Useful Addresses

Amarant Trust
80 Lambeth Road
London SE1 7PW
Tel: 020 7401 3855
Helpline: 01293 413000
www.amarantmenopausetrust.org.uk
Provides information on HRT and runs a private clinic.

British Association for Nutritional Therapy
27 Old Gloucester Street
London WC1N 3XX
Tel: 08706 061284
www.bant.org.uk
Professional body that gives advice on how to find a nutritional therapist in your area or train as one.

The Daisy Network
PO Box 183
Rossendale BB4 6WZ
Email: info@daisynetwork.org.uk
www.daisynetwork.org.uk
Support group for women with premature menopause.

Institute for Complementary Medicine
PO Box 194
London SE16 7QZ
Tel: 020 7237 5165
www.i-c-m.org.uk
Offers information and British register of accredited practitioners and recommends approved training courses.

King's Menopause Clinic
Suite 8, Golden Jubilee Wing
King's College Hospital
Denmark Hill
London SE5 9RS
Tel: 020 7346 8251
Email: hazel.mason@kingsch.nhs.uk
Menopause clinic in London open to women from outside the area.

The Menopause Exchange
PO Box 205
Bushey
Herts WD23 1ZS
Email: norma@menopause-exchange.co.uk
Organisation offering publications and advice to members.

Menopause Matters
Email: info@menopausematters.co.uk
www.menopausematters.co.uk
Independent clinician-led website providing accurate information about the menopause and its treatment options.

National Centre for Eating Disorders
54 New Road
Esher
Surrey KT10 9NU
Tel: 0845 838 2040
www.eating-disorders.org.uk

Natural Health Advisory Service
PO Box 268
Lewes
East Sussex BN7 1QN
Tel: 01273 609699
www.naturalhealthas.com

Vegan Society
Donald Watson House
21 Hylton Street
Hockley
Birmingham B18
Tel: 0121 523 1730
www.vegansociety.com

Vegetarian Society
Parkdale
Dunham Road
Altrincham
Cheshire WA14 4QG
Tel: 0161 925 2000
www.vegsoc.org

Women's Health Concern
Whitehall House
41 Whitehall
London SW1A 2BY
Tel: 0845 1232319
www.womens-health-concern.org
Offers information, advice and counselling to women with
gynaecological and hormonal problems. Publishes books and
fact sheets.

United States

American Menopause Foundation
350 Fifth Avenue, Suite 2822
New York, NY 10118
www.americanmenopause.org
Independent organisation dedicated to providing support and assistance to all issues concerning the menopause. Through a newsletter, literature and education programmes, the foundation provides the latest information on research and other facts about menopause.

The North America Menopause Society
PO Box 94527
Cleveland, OH 44101
Tel: 440 442 7550
www.menopause.org
Non-profit scientific organisation devoted to promoting understanding of menopause and improving the health of women at midlife and beyond.

US Department of Agriculture Food and Nutrition Information Center
National Agriculture Library, Room 105
1031 Baltimore Avenue
Beltsville, MD 20705
Tel: 301 504 5414

Scientific References

Chapter 1

Arnold, E. 'A voice of their own: women moving into their fifties.' *Health Care Women Int.* 2005 Sep;26(8):630-51

Stirzypulec, V. et al 'Evaluation of the quality of life of women in the climacteric period.' *Ginekol Pol.* 2004 May;75(5):373-81

Baird, D. 'Negotiating the maze: the meaning of perimenopause.' *N J Nurse.* 2004 May-Jun;34(4):17-24

Schlinder, A. E. 'Climacteric symptoms and hormones.' *Gynecol Endocrinol.* 2006 Mar;22(3):151-4

Chapter 2

Sites, C. K. 'The effect of hormone replacement therapy on body composition, body fat distribution, and insulin sensitivity in menopausal women: a randomized, double-blind, placebo-controlled trial.'

Lovejoy, J. C. 'The menopause and obesity.' *Prim Care.* 2003 Jun;30(2):317-25

Astrup, A. 'Physical activity and weight gain and fat distribution changes with menopause: current evidence and research issues.' *Med Sci Sports Exerc.* 1999 Nov;31(11 Suppl):S564-7

Simon, T. 'Why is cardiovascular health important in menopausal women?' *Climacteric.* 2006 Sep;9(5):13-8

Eliassen, A. H. et al 'Adult weight change and risk of postmenopausal breast cancer.' *JAMA.* 2006 Jul 12;296(2):193-201

Derk, C. T. 'Osteoporosis in premenopause. When are screening and treatment prudent?' *Postgrad Med.* 2006 Jun-Jul;119(1):8-15

Castelo-Branco, C. et al 'Management of menopause.' *Minerva Ginecol.* 2006 Apr;58(2):137-52

Chapter 3

Amagai, Y. et al 'Age at menopause and mortality in Japan: the Jichi Medical School Cohort Study.' *J Epidemiol.* 2006 Jul;16(4):161-6

Cassidy, A. 'Potential risks and benefits of phytoestrogen-rich diets.' *Int J Vitam Nutr Res.* 2003 Mar;73(2):120-6

Miguel, J. et al 'Menopause: A review on the role of oxygen stress and favourable effects of dietary antioxidants.' *Arch Gerontol Geriatr.* 2006 Jan 25

Wood, C. et al 'Dietary soy isoflavones inhibit estrogen effects in the postmenopausal breast.' *Cancer Res.* 2006 Jan 15;66(2):1241-9

Prentice, R. et al 'Low-fat dietary pattern and risk of invasive breast cancer: the Women's Health Initiative Randomized Controlled Dietary Modification Trial.' *JAMA.* 2006 Feb 8;295(6):629-42

Koebnick, C. et al 'The acceptability of isoflavones as a treatment of menopausal symptoms: a European survey among postmenopausal women.' *Climacteric.* 2005 Sep;8(3):230-42

Husband, A. 'Phytoestrogens and menopause. Published evidence supports a role for phytoestrogens in menopause.' *BMJ.* 2002 Jan 5;324(7328):52

Velie, E. M. et al 'Empirically derived dietary patterns and risk of postmenopausal breast cancer in a large prospective cohort study.' *Am J Clin Nutr.* 2005 Dec;82(6):1308-19

Shireffs, S. M. et al 'The effects of fluid restriction on hydration status and subjective feelings.' *Br J Nutr.* 2004 Jun;91(6):951-8

de Castro, J. M. 'The time of day of food intake influences overall intake in humans.' *J Nutr.* 2004 Jan;134(1):104-11

Drummond, S. et al 'A critique of the effects of snacking on body weight status.' *Eur J Clin Nutr.* 1996 Dec;50(12):779-83

Hatel, K. et al 'Digestive stimulant action of spices: a myth or reality?' *Indian J Med Res.* 2004 May;119(5):167-79

Leyeune, M. P. et al 'Additional protein intake limits weight regain after weight loss in humans.' *Br J Nutr.* 2005 Feb;93(2):281-9

Rolls, B. et al 'What can intervention studies tell us about the relationship between fruit and vegetable consumption and weight management?' *Nutr Rev.* 2004 Jan;62(1):1-17

Bendelius, S. 'Breakfast: is it worth it?' *School Nurse News.* 2004 Nov;21(5):16-7

Alfhag, K. et al 'Who succeeds in maintaining weight loss? A conceptual review of factors associated with weight loss maintenance and weight regain.' *Obes Rev.* 2005 Feb;6(1):67-85

Nagel, S. et al 'Reproductive and dietary determinants of the age at menopause in EPIC-Heidelberg.' *Maturitas.* 2005 Nov-Dec;52(3-4):337-47. Epub 2005 Jul 11

Robitaille, S. et al 'Effect of an oat bran-rich supplement on the metabolic profile of overweight premenopausal women.' *Ann Nutr Metab.* 2005 May-Jun;49(3):141-8. Epub 2005 May 24

Saldeen, P. et al 'Women and omega-3 fatty acids.' *Obstet Gynecol Surv.* 2004 Oct;59(10):722-30

Chapter 4

http://www.senseaboutscience.org.uk/
Chemical scientists' criticism of the detox industry is part of a 16-page report from a working group and wider consultation, published on 26 January 2006. The report challenges six major misconceptions about chemicals that pervade the lifestyle market and commentary.

Starek, A. 'Estrogens and organochlorine xenoestrogens and breast cancer risk.' *Int J Occup Med Environ Health.* 2003;16(2):113-24

Oxobia, M.N. et al 'Epidemiological risk factors for breast cancer – a review.' *Niger J Clin Pract.* 2005 Jun;8(9):35-42

Johnstone, K.L. et al 'Coffee acutely modifies gastrointestinal hormone secretion and glucose tolerance in humans: glycemic effects of chlorogenic acid and caffeine.' *Am J Clin Nutr.* 2003 Oct;78(4):728-33

Curtis, K.M. et al 'Effects of cigarette smoking, caffeine consumption, and alcohol intake on fecundability.' *Am J Epidemiol.* 1997 Jul 1;146(1):32-41

Agardh, E.E. et al 'Coffee consumption, type 2 diabetes and impaired glucose tolerance in Swedish men and women.' *J Intern Med.* 2004 Jun;255(6):645-52

Kroenkie, E. et al 'A cross-sectional study of alcohol consumption patterns and biologic markers of glycemic control among 459 women.' *Diabetes Care.* 2003 Jul;26(7):1971-8

Ropstad, E. et al 'Endocrine disruption induced by organochlorines (OCs): field studies and experimental models.' *J Toxicol Environ Health A.* 2006 Jan;69(1):53-76

Ibarreta, D. 'Possible health impact of phytoestrogens and xenoestrogens in food.' *APMIS.* 2001 Mar;109(3):161-84

Friends of the Earth press briefing for safer chemicals campaign: Chemicals and Health http://www.foe.co.uk/ campaigns/ safer_chemicals/issues/health_threats/index.html

Sirakov, M. 'Xenoestrogens – danger for the future generations?' *Akush Ginekol (Sofiia)*. 2004;43(4):39-45

Singleton, D. et al 'Xenoestrogen exposure and mechanisms of endocrine disruption.' *Front Biosci.* 2003 Jan 1;8:s110-8.

http://news.bbc.co.uk/1/hi/uk/1877162.stm

Epel, E. et al 'Stress and body shape: stress-induced cortisol secretion is consistently greater among women with central fat.' *Psychosom Med.* 2000 Sep-Oct;62(5):623-32

Epel, E. et al 'Stress may add bite to appetite in women: a laboratory study of stress-induced cortisol and eating behaviour.' *Psychoneuroendocrinology.* 2001 Jan;26(1):37-49

Chapter 6

Evans, G. et al 'Composition and biological activity of chromium-pyridine carbosyalte complexes.' *J of Inorganic Biochemistry.* 1993;49:177-87

No authors listed 'American Diabetics Association magnesium supplementation in the treatment of diabetes.' *Diabetes Care.* 1992;15:1065-7

Chasens, E. et al 'Insulin resistance and obstructive sleep apnea: is increased sympathetic stimulation the link?' *Biol Res Nurs.* 2003 Oct;5(2):87-96

Boschmann, M. et al 'Water-induced Thermogenesis.' *Journal of Clinical Endocrinology & Metabolism.* 2003; 88(12):6015-6019

Kleiner, S. 'Water: an essential but overlooked nutrient.' *J Am Diet Assoc.* 1999 Feb;99(2):200-6

Stoeckli, R. et al 'Nutritional fats and the risk of type 2 diabetes and cancer.' *Physiol Behav.* 2004 Dec 30;83(4):611-5

Tian, W. 'Weight reduction by Chinese medicinal herbs may be related to inhibition of fatty acid synthase.' *Life Sci.* 2004 Mar 26;74(19):2389-99

Preuss, H. et al 'Citrus aurantium as a thermogenic, weight-reduction replacement for ephedra: an overview.' *J Med.* 2002;33(1-4):247-64. Review

Matzkies, F. et al 'Effect of a fiber-containing dietary formula on metabolism.' *Fortschr Med.* 1982 May 20;100(19):917-20

Schrager, S. 'Dietary calcium intake and obesity.' *J Am Board Fam Pract.* 2005 May-Jun;18(3):205-10

Ipatova, O. et al 'Biological effects of the soybean phospholipids.'

Biomed Khim. 2004 Sep-Oct;50(5):436-50

Labayen, I. 'Effects of protein vs. carbohydrate-rich diets on fuel utilisation in obese women during weight loss.' *Forum Nutr.* 2003;56:168-70

Katz, D. et al 'Oats, antioxidants and endothelial function in over-weight, dyslipidemic adults.' *J Am Coll Nutr.* 2004 Oct;23(5):397-403

Roberts, D.C. et al 'The cholesterol-lowering effect of a breakfast cereal containing psyllium fibre.' *Med J Aust.* 1994 Dec 5-19;161(11-12):660-4

Elkoyam, A. et al 'The effects of allicin on weight in fructose-induced hyperinsulinemic, hyperlipidemic, hypertensive rats.' *Am J Hypertens.* 2003 Dec;16(12):1053-6

Himaya, A. et al 'The effect of soup on satiation.' *Appetite.* 1998 Apr;30(2):199-210

Morena, D. et al 'Inhibitory effects of grape seed extract on lipases.' *Nutrition.* 2003 Oct;19(10):876-9

Conceicao de Oliveira, M. et al 'Weight loss associated with a daily intake of three apples or three pears among overweight women.' *Nutrition.* 2003 Mar;19(3):253-6

Hensrud, D.D. 'Diet and obesity.' *Curr Opin Gastroenterol.* 2004 Mar;20(2):119-24

Lejeune, M.P. et al 'Effect of capsaicin on substrate oxidation and weight maintenance after modest body-weight loss in human subjects.' *Br J Nutr.* 2003 Sep;90(3):651-59

Fredrikson, G. et al 'Association between diet, lifestyle, metabolic cardiovascular risk factors, and plasma C-reactive protein levels.' *Metabolism.* 2004 Nov;53(11):1436-42

Stonge, M.P. 'Dietary fats, teas, dairy, and nuts: potential functional foods for weight control?' *Am J Clin Nutr.* 2005 Jan;81(1):7-15

Hollis, J. et al 'The effects of almond consumption on body-weight in adult females.' Purdue University, 700 W State Street, West Lafayette, IN, 47906. Paper presented at the 2005 Experimental Biology Conference, San Diego, California, April 2-6 2005

Tapsell, L. et al 'Including walnuts in a low-fat/modified-fat diet improves HDL cholesterol-to-total cholesterol ratios in patients with type 2 diabetes.' *Diabetes Care.* 2004 Dec;27(12):2777-83

Nassar, J. et al 'Calcium and magnesium ATPase activities in women with varying BMIs.' *Obes Res.* 2004 Nov;12(11):1844-50

No author listed 'Sunflower Seeds: A phytochemical Powerhouse.' National Sunflower Association, May 14, 2001/Rodriguez M. et al:

'Nutritive value of high-oleic acid sunflower seed for broiler chickens.' *Poult Sci.* 2005 Mar;84(3):395-402

Liner, E. 'Long-term efficacy of medical treatments of obesity.' *Klin Wochenschr.* 1982 Feb 1;60(3):115-20

Kingston, R. et al 'The relative safety of ephedra compared with other herbal products.' *Ann Intern Med.* 2003 Mar 18;138(6):468-71

Gonzalez, M. et al 'Effect of a dietary supplement combination on weight management, adipose tissue, cholesterol and triglycerides in obese subjects.' *P R Health Sci J.* 2004 Jun;23(2):121-4

Heber, D. 'Herbal preparations for obesity: are they useful?' *Prim Care.* 2003 Jun;30(2):441-63

McMillan, T. et al 'Complementary and alternative medicine and physical activity for menopausal symptoms.' *J Am Med Women's Assoc.* 2004 Fall;59(4):270-7

Dobnov, G. et al 'Weight control and the management of obesity after menopause: the role of physical activity.' *Maturitas.* 2003 Feb 25;44(2):89-101

Kruger, J. et al 'Dietary and physical activity behaviors among adults successful at weight loss maintenance.' *Int J Behav Nutr Phys Act.* 2006 Jul 19;3:17

Chapter 7

Cook, A. et al 'Phytoestrogen and multiple vitamin/mineral effects on bone mineral density in early postmenopausal women: a pilot study.' *J Womens Health Gend Based Med.* 2002 Jan-Feb;11(1):53-60

Albertazzi, P. et al 'The effect of dietary soy supplementation on hot flushes.' *Obstet Gynecol.* 1998;91:6-11

Komesarrott, P. et al 'Effects of wild yam extract on menopausal symptoms, lipids and sex hormones in healthy menopausal women.' *Climacteric.* 2001 Jun;4(2):144-50

Kronenberg, F. et al 'Complementary and alternative medicine for menopausal symptoms: a review of randomized, controlled trials.' *Ann Intern Med.* 2002 Nov 19;137(10):805-13

Fitzpatrick, L. 'Alternatives to estrogen.' *Med Clin North Am.* 2003;87(5):1091-113

Gass, M. 'Alternatives for women through menopause.' *Am J Obstet Gynecol.* 2001;185(2 Suppl):S47-56

Israel, D. et al 'Herbal therapies for perimenopausal and menopausal complaints.' *Pharmacotherapy.* 1997;17:970-84

Morelli, V. et al 'Alternative therapies for traditional disease states: menopause.' *Am Fam Physician*. 2002;66(1):129-34

Tesch, B. 'Herbs commonly used by women: an evidence-based review.' *Am J Obstet Gynecol*. 2003;188(5 Suppl):S44-55

Geller, S. et al 'Botanical and dietary supplements for menopausal symptoms: what works, what does not.' *J Women's Health (Larchmt)*. 2005 Sep;14(7):634-49

Beattie, J. et al 'The influence of a low-boron diet and boron supplementation on bone, major mineral and sex steroid metabolism in postmenopausal women.' *Br J Nutr*. 1993 May;69(3):871-84

Ilich, J.Z. 'A lighter side of calcium: role of calcium and dairy foods in body weight.' *Arh Hig Rada Toksikol*. 2005 Mar;56(1):33-8

Daniele, C. et al 'Vitex agnus castus: a systematic review of adverse events.' *Drug Saf*. 2005;28(4):319-32

Chapter 8

Balch, J.F. and Balch, P. *Prescription for Nutritional Healing*. Garden City Park, NY: Avery Publishing Group, 1997. ISBN 0-89529-727-2

Brandt, K.D. 'Effects of nonsteroidal anti-inflammatory drugs on chondrocyte metabolism in vitro and in vivo.' *Am J Med*. 1987;83(5A):29-34

Brooks, P.M., Potter, S.R. and Buchanan, W.W. 'NSAID and osteoarthritis – help or hindrance?' *J Rheumatol*. 1982;9:3-5

Brown, Donald J. 'Vitex agnus castus. Clinical Monograph.' *Quarterly Review of Natural Medicine*. Summer 1994: 111-120

Burton, A.F. and Anderson, F.H. 'Decreased incorporation of 14C-glucosamine relative to 3H-N-acetylglucosamine in the intestinal mucosa of patients with inflammatory bowel disease.' *Am J Gastroenterol*. 1983;78:19-22

Capps, J.C. et al. 'Hexosamine metabolism II. Effect of insulin and phlorizin on the absorption and metabolism, in vivo, of D-glucosamine and N-acetyl-glucosamine in the rat.' *Biochim Biophys Acta*. 1966;127:205-12

Carper, J. *The Food Pharmacy*. New York, NY: Bantam Books, 1988

Capps, J.C. and Shetlar, M.R. 'In vivo incorporation of D-glucosamine I-C14 into acid mucopolysaccharides of rabbit liver.' *Proc Soc Expot Biol Med*. 1963;114:118-20

Davis, Patricia. *Aromatherapy: an A-Z*. Saffron Walden, England:

C.W. Daniel Company Limited, 1995. ISBN 0-85207-295-3

Drovanti, A. et al. 'Therapeutic activity of oral glucosamine sulfate in osteoarthrosis: a placebo-controlled double-blind investigation.' *Clin Ther.* 1980;3:260-72

Fulder, S. and Blackwood, J. *Garlic, Nature's Original Remedy.* Rochester, Vermont: Healing Arts Press, 1991. ISBN 0-89281-436-5

Hendler, S.S. *The Doctors' Vitamin and Mineral Encyclopedia.* New York, NY: Simon and Schuster, 1990. ISBN 0-671-66784-X

Hoffman, David. *The Complete Illustrated Holistic Herbal.* Shaftesbury, Dorset: Element Books, 1996. ISBN 1-85230-847-8

Horvilleur, A. *The Family Guide to Homeopathy.* Virginia: Health and Homeopathy Publishing Inc., 1986. ISBN 0-9616800-0-8

Kohn, P. et al. 'Metabolism of D-glucosamine and N-acetyl-D-glucosamine in the intact rat.' *J Biol Chem* 237:304-8, 1962

Lark, Susan M. *The Menopause Self Help Book.* Berkeley, CA: Celestial Arts, 1990. ISBN 0-89087-592-8

Lark, Susan M. *Women's Health Companion Self-Help Nutrition Guide and Cookbook.* Berkeley, CA: Celestial Arts, 1995, paperback 1996. ISBN 0-89087-733-5

Morrison, M. 'Therapeutic applications of chondroitin-4-sulfate, appraisal of biologic properties.' *Folia Angiol.* 1977;25:225-32

Murray, Michael. *5-HTP, the Natural Way to Overcome Depression, Obesity, and Insomnia.* New York, NY: Bantam Books, 1998. ISBN 0-533-19784-4

Murray, Michael. 'Glucosamine sulfate: Effective osteoarthritis treatment.' *The American Journal of Natural Medicine.* 1994 Sept;1(1)

Murray, Michael T. *Menopause: How to Benefit From Diet, Vitamins, Minerals, Herbs and Other Natural Methods.* Prima Publishing, 1994. ISBN 1559584270

Newman, N.M. and Ling, R.S. 'Acetabular bone destruction related to non-steroidal anti-inflammatory drugs.' *Lancet.* 1985;2:11-13

Peirce, A. *The American Pharmaceutical Association Practical Guide to Natural Medicines.* New York, NY: Stonesong Press, 1999. ISBN 0-688-16151-0

Pujalte, J.M. et al. 'Double-blind clinical evaluation of oral glucosamine sulphate in the basic treatment of osteoarthritis.' *Curr Med Res Opin.* 1980;7:110-4

Ronningen, H. and Langeland, N. 'Indomethacin treatment in osteoarthritis of the hip joint.' *Acta Orthop Scand.* 1979;50:169-74

Setnikar, I. et al. 'Antiarthritic effects of glucosamine sulfate studied in animal models.' *Arzneimittelforschung.* 1991; 41:542-5

Shield, M.J. 'Anti-inflammatory drugs and their effects on cartilage synthesis and renal function.' *Eur J Rhematol Inflam.* 1993;13:7-16

Solomon, L. 'Drug induced arthropathy and necrosis of the femoral head.' *Journal Bone Joint Surg.* 1973;55B: 246-51

Tesoriere, G. et al. 'Intestinal absorption of glucosamine and N-acetylglucosamine.' *Experientia.* 1972;28-770-1

Vliet, Elizabeth L. *Screaming to be Heard, Hormonal Connections Women Suspect and Doctors Ignore.* New York, NY: M. Evans and Company, Inc., 1995. ISBN 0-87131-784-2

Weed, Susan. *Menopausal Years: The Wise Woman Way – Alternative Approaches for Women 30–90.* Woodstock, New York: Ash Tree, 1992. ISBN 9614620-4-3

Weil, A. *Eating Well for Optimum Health.* New York: Alfred A. Knopf, 2000. ISBN 0-375-40754-5

Willard, Terry. *Textbook of Advanced Herbology.* Calgary: CW Progressive Publishing Inc., 1992. ISBN 0-9691727-1-0

Willard, Terry. *Textbook of Modern Herbology* (rev. 2nd ed.). Calgary: CW Progressive Publishing Inc., 1993. ISBN 0-9691727-4-5

Willard, Terry. *The Wild Rose Scientific Herbal.* Calgary: Wild Rose College of Natural Healing, Ltd. 1st hardcover 1991; 2nd printing 1998. ISBN 0-9691727-0-3

Yoshiro, K. 'The Physiological actions of tang-kuei and cnidium.' *Bull Oriental Healing Arts Inst USA* 1985;10:269-78

'Treatment of High Blood Pressure.' National Heart, Lung, and Blood Institute. Available at: http://www.nhlbi.nih.gov /hbp/treat/treat.htm. Accessed 5 May 2006

'Complementary and alternative medicine and physical activity for menopausal symptoms.' *J Am Med Women's Assoc.* 2004 Fall;59(4):270-7

'Nonhormonal therapies for hot flashes in menopause.' *Am Fam Physician.* 2006 Feb 1;73(3):457-64

Nedrow, A. et al 'Complementary and alternative therapies for the management of menopause-related symptoms: a systematic evidence review.' *Arch Intern Med.* 2006 Jul 24;166(14):1453-65

Dailey, K. et al 'Herbal product use and menopause symptom relief in primary care patients: a MetroNet study.' *J Women's Health (Larchmt).* 2003 Sep;12(7):633-41

Tiran, D. 'Integrated healthcare: herbal remedies for menopausal symptoms.' *Br J Nurs.* 2006 Jun 22-Jul 12;15(12):645-8

Swanson, J. et al 'Urinary incontinence: common problem among women over 45.' *Can Fam Physician.* 2005 Jan;51:84-5

Chan, M. et al 'Osteoporosis prevention education programme for women.' *J Adv Nurs.* 2006 Apr;54(2):159-70

Walker, A.R. 'Breast cancer – can risks really be lessened?' *Eur J Cancer Prev.* 2000 Aug;9(4):223-9

Arias, R.D. 'Cardiovascular health and the menopause: the gynecologist as the patients' interface.' *Climacteric.* 2006 Sep;9(5):6-12

Hu, F.B. 'Overweight and obesity in women: health risks and consequences.' *J Women's Health (Larchmt).* 2003 Mar;12(2):163-72

Chapter 9

Bakken, K. et al 'Side-effects of hormone replacement therapy and influence on pattern of use among women aged 45–64 years.' The Norwegian Women and Cancer (NOWAC) study 1997. *Acta Obstet Gynecol Scand.* 2004 Sep;83(9):850-6

Jensen, L.B. et al 'Hormone replacement therapy dissociates fat mass and bone mass, and tends to reduce weight gain in early postmenopausal women: a randomized controlled 5-year clinical trial of the Danish Osteoporosis Prevention Study.' *J Bone Miner Res.* 2003 Feb;18(2):333-42

Heikkinen, J. et al 'A 10-year follow-up of postmenopausal women on long-term continuous combined hormone replacement therapy: update of safety and quality-of-life findings.' *J Br Menopause Soc.* 2006 Sep;12(3):115-25

Watt, P. et al 'A holistic programmatic approach to natural hormone replacement.' *Fam Community Health.* 2003 Jan-Mar;26(1):53-63

Dennerstein, L. et al 'Life satisfaction, symptoms, and the menopausal transition.' *Medscape Womens Health.* 2000 Jul-Aug;5(4):E4

Addis, I.B. et al 'Sexual activity and function in middle-aged and older women.' *Obstet Gynecol.* 2006 Apr;107(4):755-64

Lindau, S.T. et al 'Older women's attitudes, behaviour, and communication about sex and HIV: a community-based study.' *J Women's Health (Larchmt).* 2006 Jul-Aug;15(6):747-53

Ball, K. et al 'Effects of cognitive training interventions with older adults: a randomized controlled trial.' *JAMA.* 2002 Nov 13;288(18):2271

INDEX